Taking Charge

Making Your Healthcare Appointments Work for You

Written by

Ricky White

Taking Charge

Making Your Healthcare Appointments Work for You

ISBN-13: 978-1541343191

ISBN-10: 1541343190

http://rickywhite.net/

Cover design by Rob Ellis.

Dedication

Katie,

You have taught me more about myself than I ever thought possible. I am better for knowing you, better for loving you, and better for giving myself to you.

I could not help people to better themselves if you hadn't bettered me, first.

This book is dedicated to you.

Always and forever.

Acknowledgements

There are many people I need to thank, without whom this book would not have made it. The task of writing a book—regardless of the topic or size—is an arduous one. It takes love and support from those closest to you. This book was no different.

To my wife, who has been my confidant, cheerleader, and moral support throughout the process of writing this book. You have been there to nag me to write when I needed it the most. And took care of me when I was too exhausted to do any more. Chronic illness and long hours *do not* go together. But you helped me through it. For that I am, as always, eternally grateful.

To Jennifer, at Magic Wand Editing (**magicwandediting.com**), your job was not an easy one. Thank you for your patience and professionalism. I hope you enjoyed reading my manuscript for the first time half as much as I did writing it.

Thank you to Cascades Photography (**http://www.cascadesphotography.com/**), for providing me with an excellent service, and excellent photographs. You even managed to get me to smile for a photo. That in itself is a remarkable achievement.

They say never judge a book by its cover. Everyone knows that's utter nonsense. Everyone does. I consider the cover for this book to be a fantastic one. Thank you, Rob Ellis. You are a talent, sir.

I would also like to give a special thanks Adrienne Taren MD PhD, Dr. Marek Parkola MBBCH, Martin Belcher, and Russ Meserve. Be proud of yourselves. Without your feedback this book might not have got this far.

And thank you to those of you who have been with me from the start. There are too many to name, I'm sorry. But that doesn't mean I'm not thankful, because I am, eternally.

Contents

CHAPTER ONE

Introduction

What is this book about?

If there is one thing in life that's inevitable, it's illness. At some point, we all get sick—whether it's temporary or long-term, it's going to happen one day. And when that day comes, we seek help from doctors and healthcare professionals who guide us down the road to better health. Well, that's the hope, at least.

Not all are so fortunate. Not everyone can get better. Chronic illnesses are rife in our society, and the best that can be hoped for is to not get any worse, as there is often no cure. In the United States, around half of all adults—117 million people—have one or more chronic health conditions, and one in four adults have two or more chronic health conditions.[1] In 2012, there were over 928 million physician visits in the United States, with over half of those (54 percent) to primary care doctors. That equates to 300.8 visits per 100 people.[2] That's a lot of appointments!

I am one of those statistics, too. In 2010, I was diagnosed with a chronic degenerative illness called ankylosing spondylitis (also referred to as A.S.). My life changed dramatically overnight. Most of these changes I would learn to live with. And I'm still learning, to be completely honest. I probably always will be. But the part I thought would be the easiest turned out to be more challenging than I anticipated: doctors' appointments.

In the beginning, I didn't know the system. I didn't understand what it was like to be sitting on the patient's side of the desk. I thought I did, but I was blissfully unaware of just how complicated and time-consuming attending doctor's appointments can be, especially when you have to see more than one doctor or specialist.

The fact that you're reading this right now means you're probably in a similar situation. Are you exasperated with all your appointments? Do you come out of your appointments with unanswered questions, or with even more questions than before? Are you getting frustrated that your care isn't coordinated? Do you have trouble keeping track of all the changes in your care? Is there too much jargon and information? Or do you always find that you don't agree with your doctor, and that you're not on the same page?

If you answered "yes" to any of the above questions, you should definitely read on. You are the person who inspired me to write this book.

How will this book help you?

Okay, I'll be honest with you. What you will not find in this book is a magic formula or a quick fix to getting the kind of care you deserve. It just doesn't work like that. I'm sure you knew that anyway, right?

What you will find in this book is a whole group of tools to add to your toolbox. I call them tools because the strategies and methods in these pages will work the same way as the tools in your toolbox. You'll need to pick the right tool for the right job, depending on your individual needs. Because that's what you are: an individual. You are not a generic patient. You are unique, with your own problems to solve. It would be unfair and unjust of me to try to treat you otherwise.

This will be a learning process. It will take practice to implement the methods in this book effectively. But that's okay. Nothing good ever came easy, right? And I know that, despite what you might think, your doctor will appreciate the effort you put in, too. He or she (let's use "she," for this chapter) will be glad you're taking your health seriously and will be even more willing and empathetic in helping you achieve the best outcome possible, but more on that later.

As we go on, I will refer to resources which were created specifically for this book. These are FREE and can be downloaded at any time from my website. Please use them as you see fit. You won't necessarily need them all, or perhaps you won't need them today. But these tools are my gift to you, whether you need them now or years from now.

Throughout this book, I'll be referring to "your doctor" a lot, but the same principles and methods I discuss can be used for all your healthcare appointments. So regardless of whom you're seeing— a nurse, physiotherapist, occupational therapist, or other specialist—you can use the contents of this book to approach your appointment just the same. The aim of this book is to arm you with the tools you'll need for the job, and, as I said before, depending on the situation or professional you are seeing you will need to pick the appropriate tools for your needs.

Why is it important to have a good relationship with your doctors?

Because you'll get better care. It really is that simple. But let me elaborate a little.

Your relationship with your doctor is like any other. You'll get more out of it, with fewer arguments and less stress, if you have a healthy one.

All relationships are two-sided, of course, and they need both parties to put in the work. But the more willing you are to be open and honest with your doctor, the more likely she is to do the same. Doctors are people, too, and they only have so much time and energy, just like you. Next time you have a stressful day, I want you to think about what tasks you gave your time and energy to. Was there anything into which you only put in the minimal amount of effort to get the job done? It's quite likely that there were tasks you performed that day that you didn't do as well as you normally would. Doctors are no different, especially busy, overworked doctors. So, if you were the doctor, and you were running on empty, would you save your energy (often subconsciously) for the patient who doesn't seem to give a damn about you and who doesn't seem to be taking his or her health seriously? Or would you save your energy so you can give the best care to the patient who is taking his or her health seriously and who cares about you, too? I know I would, and probably did.

What I'm *not* saying is that doctors purposefully give bad care to patients they don't like. Even the few bad apples in the medical profession still care. They are not going to withhold treatment options from you just because they choose to. But if you have a good working relationship with your doctor, you are more likely to get even better care, because the small things that can be overlooked are more likely to be dealt with.

Take your health seriously—as you no doubt do; you are reading this book, after all—and your doctor will be more likely to go the extra mile for you, and that can make all the difference. It may not make any difference at all in your care, depending on your current relationship, but what's wrong with showing you care and being nice, just for the sake of doing so? Absolutely nothing at all.

Why me?

Prior to my expatriation to the United States, I lived in the United Kingdom, where I worked as a registered nurse. For the last five years of my career as a nurse (post-A.S. diagnosis), I worked in an outpatient clinic environment, where people came to see me for their appointments. This put me in the unique and advantageous position of sitting on both sides of the desk.

Being able to see things from both the patient's and the healthcare professional's view gave me an understanding that most don't have. I was able to enter my own appointments with a different perspective, and, more importantly, with the knowledge of what my doctors wanted from me and how best to present it. Being an "insider" gave me an advantage when it came to getting the correct care. It shouldn't be that way. I'm not saying I was treated better because I was a nurse; that wasn't the case. But being able to make the best use of my 10-15-minute appointment without wasting time, and without leaving with unanswered questions, meant my care was far more streamlined.

Now not all my appointments went swimmingly. But would you trust me if I said they did? Of course not; I wouldn't. Even with my "insider" knowledge, I've made mistakes. But I've learned from them. This book is just as much as about learning from your mistakes as it is about learning how to approach and conduct your appointments. But we'll cover all that in the later chapters.

For now, just be assured that I understand your frustrations, and I'm here to share my knowledge as a healthcare professional *and* as a patient.

CHAPTER TWO

Barriers

What is a barrier, and why does it matter?

A barrier is simply anything that is stopping you from communicating effectively with your doctor, which then has an impact on the care you receive. The barrier(s) will be personal to you. I can only guide you to finding them; you have to do the hard work and figure out what your barriers are. Sorry.

Once you have identified your barrier(s), you will be able to plan your appointments more effectively, because you will know what you need to focus on. This will enable you to pick the appropriate tools for the job, so that you can break down your barriers and start to strengthen the relationship between you and your doctor. We'll cover specifically how to do that later in this book.

It's also important to note that you might, and most likely will, have different barriers with different doctors and specialists. Don't assume the same approach will work each time. You'll need to identify your barriers individually and make a plan of action for each in turn. Thankfully, this shouldn't be something you need to do every time you have a doctor's appointment if you address it early on. It may not, however, be an easy fix, and may take some time and effort to break down your barriers.

Some of these barriers will be obvious. If they are, great. You may already be working on them. Sometimes we (as patients) are causing the barrier, and that can be hard to admit to ourselves. So let's run through a few common barriers that I have encountered in my experience sitting on both sides of the desk. This is not an exhaustive list by any measure, but having an idea will help you start to identify your own barriers. I will help you acquire the tools you need to address these in the "Planning" and "Communication" chapters of this book later. So for now, make a note of your own barriers so that we can address them later, when you know how.

Jargon

Let's warm up with an easy one. Is the barrier simply that you don't understand what is being said to you? Lots of long words that seem impossible to spell? I've been there—try spelling "ankylosing spondylitis" for the first time. Even as a nurse, I needed to look up some of the jargon I came across, or the special scoring system the doctor used, after my appointments, just so I could better understand what was said. You should, too. Don't be afraid to ask your doctor to clarify things. Sometimes just saying, "I'm sorry, I don't understand; could you go over that again, please?" is necessary.

Physical barriers

Are you traveling to a healthcare appointment that is somewhere you've never been? Is there adequate parking? Do you have a long way to walk once you get there? If so, can you do it? Is there public transport close by, and do you know which stop you need? Will you need to fast today for your bloods tests? If so, is there somewhere you can eat afterwards? Physical barriers are very common, and often anxiety-inducing when you don't have the answers. Thankfully, with a little planning they are usually one of the easier problems on this list to solve.

Time

Sometimes you have more than one medical appointment in one day. Other times you might have to get back to collect the kids from childcare or school. Maybe there's an important meeting you just can't miss. Whatever your own activities are, you only have twenty-four hours in the day to achieve them, and it's never enough. Be conscious of time. If you plan correctly, nothing need be missed.

Anxiety/nervousness

I have no statistics to back this up, so this is just my own opinion, but getting anxious and nervous at appointments seems to happen quite frequently, more so than I used to imagine. Sometimes this can stop you from thinking clearly, or maybe you just forget what was said because you were worrying about something else instead. Don't be embarrassed or disheartened if this is you. Recognizing it is half of the battle. How you deal with this depends on the cause of your anxiety or nervousness. Maybe you are anxious because you are not sure what to expect? Or are you nervous because you don't know where you need to go? These are barriers that can be, in part, addressed with good planning. If this is you, be sure to make good use of the "Planning" chapter later on.

Emotional barriers and taboo

If you can't tell your doctor your embarrassing problem or circumstance, who can you tell it to? Maybe in your culture or religion certain things are taboo. But when you're with your doctor, you need to try to push those uncomfortable feelings aside and discuss the issues anyway. You won't get the care you deserve by shying away from certain issues.

Also, please don't be embarrassed if your emotions get the best of you. If you've just been given bad news, you've had a recent loss in the family, or you are having marital problems, that's okay. You aren't going to be able to put those emotions to one side and forget about them—they're too strong. Nor should you. But if you mention to your doctor why you are in your current mood, it will help him (and we'll use "him" for this chapter, and keep alternating) understand you and your circumstances and help him guide the rest of the appointment appropriately. Don't think of your emotions as an excuse, but as more of a condition of being human.

Aiming for different goals

This is quite an important barrier to break down. You will never get to where you want to go if you and your doctor are driving in different directions. You both need to be on the same page. Most of the time people don't realize that their doctor's goals may be different from their own, and that may well be because of poor communication. It's important to make sure you're shooting for the same goal(s). If you're not sure, you need to ask your doctor what he honestly hopes to achieve.

Lack of confidence

Sometimes you have to be proactive in your approach to better care. You may need the confidence to ask questions like "Why?", "What are the side effects?", "Is there an alternative?", or "What happens if this treatment fails?" All of these are perfectly simple and expected questions that, frankly, you shouldn't have to ask. But you may need to. To do so—to question someone else—takes confidence. We aren't all confident, and if you are, you may not be in this situation. If the ability to speak up and to question is a barrier for you, then the "Effective Communication" chapter may be the most useful for you.

Money/insurance

In my opinion, it's unfortunate that money plays a part in healthcare, period. But it does. Even if you live in a country like the United Kingdom, where healthcare is free at the point of contact and comes at no cost to the patient, there are still money implications behind the scenes. Sometimes this means that a particular treatment is not available because it is not considered "cost effective." This happened to me *twice*. I was refused a drug (etanercept) that could have helped me. It was even recommended by the National Institute for Health and Care Excellence, but because I had tried a similar drug already and "failed," I was refused funding for the new treatment. My Primary Care Trust (the NHS body that supplies funding) had no legal obligation to provide it for me. When I moved, I fell under a different Primary Care Trust, so naturally, I reapplied. I was refused again, for the same reason. So even in a country with free healthcare, there are limitations.

The same situations occur in the United States, too. If your insurance doesn't cover a treatment, then you don't get it unless you pay for it yourself. It's sad that this happens.

So what can be done about this barrier? Unfortunately, very little. If you're in the United Kingdom, you could move to a different area and try your luck at the infamous "postcode lottery," but this is unlikely to be a practical solution. Instead, you will need to have some serious discussions with your doctor about your plan B. If you're in the United States and your insurance doesn't cover your treatment, you may find that there are ways of paying for all or part of it without furthering your own medical expenses, as there are a number of programs and charities that offer funding for certain treatments. The problem is that your doctor is unlikely to know about them, and certainly not all of them, so you have to do the research and legwork yourself. You will have to meet certain criteria to qualify, but if you're in a low-income family, you will almost certainly qualify. These charities and schemes can also be region-specific, so you may need to check drug company and local websites for information.

Personal barriers

Have you ever had a conversation with someone, only to realize afterward that you barely paid attention and can't quite remember what was said because you were either distracted or disengaged? I have. I'm pretty sure everyone has at some point. If this happens when you're sitting with a healthcare professional, it could have serious implications, or, at best, you'll leave the appointment feeling like it was a waste of time.

So why were you disengaged? Did you get a bad first impression? This is almost certainly going to start your relationship with your doctor on the wrong foot. First impressions count. If they're bad, you need to try and look past that if you're going to have a productive appointment. If it was because the doctor didn't wash his hands before or after doing your exam, then you should speak up about it. That's a problem that can be addressed. If it was because the doctor looked disheveled, there is little you can do unless personal hygiene is a factor, in which case a complaint may be warranted. Was it because your doctor's accent was hard to understand? Then ask for clarification.

The other personal barrier I have come across is a big one, and is hard to rectify at times. That is the barrier of a closed mind.

In order to get the best and appropriate care for you, you have to make *informed* decisions. Closing your mind to other possibilities restricts you immensely. It is impossible to make an informed decision about your own care if you don't know about alternative treatments—which even include the "do nothing" option. By going to your appointment with blinders on, you may be setting yourself up to choose the wrong treatment option. If you take the time to listen to all the options from your doctor, he will in turn listen to your suggestion(s), too. But don't be closed-minded, and respectfully discuss all options. Regardless of what your decision is, make sure it is an informed one.

CHAPTER THREE

What Doctors Expect From You

This book wouldn't be complete without looking at the expectations doctors and other healthcare professionals have of you, the patient. Knowing what they expect will enable you to approach the appointment more appropriately and will help guide your pre-appointment planning.

Without further ado, here is a breakdown of some of the important things to remember during your appointment:

Be honest and tell your doctor everything

This might sound obvious, but many people still don't tell the truth for many reasons. Medicine is a research-based practice. This means that doctors like facts. Lies don't cut it, and they could have serious implications for your treatment options and health. Most lies from patients aren't deliberate or malicious, and in my experience, they often are used to hide embarrassment. So let's get one thing straight: Your doctor has probably heard it before, and if not, she isn't going to be surprised. It's understandable to get embarrassed about things—we all do. But as a patient, you have the legal right to confidentiality. No one else need know, if that is your wish. Just have some common sense. Don't take your spouse with you to the appointment if you think your girlfriend or boyfriend on-the-side has given you an STD and you don't want your spouse finding out. Doctors can't treat stupid. (And yes, that actually happened.)

Being honest doesn't just apply to your symptoms or your situation, either. If I had a buck for every time a patient "forgot to mention" something they were taking, I wouldn't need to write this book. And I'm not just talking about booze and illegal drugs. If you've been taking Viagra, but you don't want your wife to know because you're embarrassed and she's sitting next to you, tough luck. Tell your doctor, either before the appointment or at the appointment, but *not* after.

You may just think those nutritional or creatine

supplements are harmless. I mean, you're in much better shape now, right? They may well affect your blood work, altering your treatment. The same goes for those herbal supplements and homeopathic treatments. And don't assume that just because you bought it over the counter at a pharmacy, it doesn't matter and it's safe. Some herbal remedies have blood-thinning effects; did you know that? This is particularly important if you need surgery.

If there is just one thing you take away from this book, I hope it is to be honest with yourself and with your doctor. You can't expect good and appropriate care from your medical team if they don't have all the facts. No matter how unimportant or unrelated you may think something is, it doesn't matter; it could be vital to your health.

Be punctual

Another obvious one, right? Yet many are still late for appointments. The blame is often passed off as "the train was late," "my meeting ran long," or "traffic was a nightmare." In my mind, and in the mind of other healthcare professionals, these are not genuine excuses. They all come down to poor planning (and we will be covering this later in the book). If you live in a city, expect traffic to be a nightmare; it always is! Plan to catch the earlier train in case it is late. Plan for the worst. If you're late for your appointment, the person you're annoying least is probably the doctor. She has so much to do, she could fill the time, if she has no one else she can see instead. The people most annoyed are the other patients. If you're late, then other people's appointments following yours are late, too. Have you been in the situation where others have been late and you spend ages in the waiting room because of it? It's one of the most frustrating things there is. Don't be that person.

Okay, so the elephant in the room—let's get it out of the way. I know what some of you are thinking: "But doctors always run late, so why be there early just to wait around longer?" I'm not going to bore you with all the intricacies of this issue—that would be a whole new book—but I do want to address briefly a few points regarding this:

- Being late purposefully because you think you'll save yourself some time actually compounds the issue. There is a team of staff helping with your appointment today, not just a doctor. Some of these people you will never see or meet, but they are there, trust me. The doctor is usually the last, or the last but one, person in the chain. Any delay to any of the preceding people ultimately leads you to waiting for the doctor.

- Rarely does a clinic run late because the doctor is late for work. Often, doctors have other commitments to meet before they start seeing patients. They hate running late, too, as do all the other members of the team.

Providing all patients arrived on time, doctors tend to run behind schedule for one of two reasons:

Firstly, there are too many patients scheduled in that day. The word all healthcare professionals hate to hear or see is "overbooked." It may surprise you to hear that both in the United Kingdom and in the United States, doctors have little to no control over how many patients they see a day. Their clinics are almost always controlled by the management of the healthcare provider, especially in the National Health Service (NHS) in the United Kingdom. Please bear this in mind when you complain that you've been waiting over an hour. There's probably little that could have been done by the doctors, nurses, and reception staff to avoid it, so please don't take your frustration out on them personally. Instead say something along the lines of, "I'm sorry, you seem to be having a busy day, I hope you've managed to get a break. I was just wondering how much longer you anticipate the wait, as I've already been waiting over an hour, and I have to get back to work" (insert your own personal issue). A little kindness and empathy goes a long way.

Secondly, patients have complex needs, and sometimes doctors just can't address the problem in the allotted time. I've heard people say things like, "Once they get their ten minutes, they should kick them out and call the next patient." This is not helpful. And frankly, it's rather a callous attitude. In these situations, I'm keen to point out to those individuals that maybe they wouldn't feel the same way if the doctor kicked them out of the office on time, forcing them to make a second appointment to come back and address their needs. Some things just need more time. There are some people who have been dealt shitty hands in life—maybe you're one of them—and they deserve to have their problems treated with the same amount of respect as others, and not to be rushed through their appointments.

Be respectful

It's easy when you are in pain or unwell to be short and grumpy with others without good reason. That's okay; we all do it. I'm sure my wife will attest to that. Doctors understand this, too. But it makes life easier for all parties if you try not to be short and aggressive in your speech.

Respect obviously goes both ways, and you should

definitely expect the same in return. But one thing guaranteed to negatively affect your relationship with your doctor is speaking disrespectfully of other healthcare professionals, particularly if you talk about "firing" your last doctor. Now, of course, he or she may have been a bad doctor, but bad doctors aren't as common as people believe. Sometimes doctors don't get along with their patients, but that doesn't make them bad physicians, just bad communicators. As a patient, you also have the right to a second opinion, a right I implore you to use if you feel ill-informed or unsatisfied with your treatment options. But talking negatively and disrespectfully about another doctor will start you off on the wrong foot with your new doctor (or with your current doctor, if you're speaking ill of a specialist). Don't get labeled as a "troublesome patient" just because you didn't think before you spoke. And, yes, bad patients exist just as much as bad doctors, but neither exist as much as the other side thinks. Bad communication is the culprit in most cases, which is more reason to keep reading on.

Stick to the plan

One thing that I hate, both as a patient and as a healthcare professional, is the teeth-grinding phrase "non-compliant." Urgh!

I won't deny that sometimes there are valid reasons

for stopping a treatment. And, of course, it's your care, so you have the final say in what direction it takes. If you are having a reaction to a new medication or have uncontrollable side effects, then stopping is advised, but you should immediately tell your doctor that you are stopping and why. In fact, there should always be a plan B of some kind when starting a new medication. That is something that can be lacking in patient care sometimes.

I've heard the story many times. Someone is prescribed a new medication, she has a reaction or her symptoms get worse, so she stops the medication and tells her doctor at the next appointment in three months' time. That scenario happens too often. In that case, there are failings on both sides. If you are being prescribed a new medication, ask the question, "What happens if ...?" Know what is expected from you if the new medication doesn't work. Do you email or call the doctor? Do you book an urgent appointment with her first? These are things you need to consider. If the information isn't offered to you, as it should be, then ask.

The scenario above is not non-compliance. In fact, it is the opposite. It's compliance if you've followed the alternate plan, or the "What if?"

Non-compliance would be if you stopped taking a

medication, or that you didn't follow a treatment plan, such as dietary changes or weight loss, and that you didn't follow a plan B, either because you chose not to or because there wasn't one. You can't be forced to take medication you don't want or to follow a plan you don't believe in. We are all free to make our own choices based on what we think and feel is best for us. You can still achieve that while remaining compliant.

Whatever your reason for not following a treatment plan, whether "valid" or not, the issue often is one of poor communication. When both sides communicate well, not only will you both know the "why" of this treatment, but you will both be clear on when stopping might be better than carrying on. If you and your doctor are communicating well, then non-compliance may become compliance, even if the outcome is the same.

The issue of non-compliance is a long and complicated one, and I have only scratched the surface here. Not following through on plans makes it difficult to manage your condition and for you to get the right treatment. Sometimes side effects pass, and sometimes they just need to be managed better. If the treatment ends up working, then it may well be worth it to carry on despite the side effects. What annoys doctors the most is when a patient stops a medication before its efficacy has been determined. This makes effective treatment of the problem difficult for you both. Communication before starting a treatment is key to making sure that you give the treatment is given a chance, while maintaining your own expectations. It's a balance that can be difficult, which reinforces the argument for good communication on both sides.

Research carefully

Everyone loves Google. I love Google and Bing. And if you're rolling your eyes right now, we're all free to like what we like, within the limits of the law. It doesn't mean I'm weird for liking Bing. Anyway ...

Researching your problem before you see the doctor can be very helpful. Knowledge is power. But please don't be the patient who thinks a Google (or Bing) search and the handful of research articles he or she has printed is in any way a substitute for a medical degree.

Understanding the problem and how it's treated is a good thing, but it doesn't mean that a) what you found is the most appropriate course of action for you, or b) your self-diagnosis is correct in the first place. Many diseases and conditions share signs and symptoms. In fact, I'm reminded of something I learned in nursing school which I never forgot: Two patients could be lying in beds next to each other and have identical symptoms, but have two completely different problems that need completely different treatments. It's something I've encountered over and over throughout my career.

I'm going to repeat something I said earlier: You are not a generic patient. You are unique, with your own needs, so treat yourself uniquely and not as a checklist of symptoms from the internet.

I have just one thing more to say on reading and collecting research papers: New research is constantly being published, and it can be very hard for a healthcare professional to keep up. However, as a patient I would not advocate relying on these publications alone, particularly not on "new" research. Unless you have training and extensive experience in academically critiquing medical research, it will be difficult to judge whether what you have in your hands is "good" research. Showing such research to your doctor may have a negative impact on your relationship, and it will extend the length of your appointment because your doctor may have to explain why it is not reliable research, which is counterproductive. Also, even if you find multiple articles that come to the same conclusion, that doesn't mean the findings are true. Why? Because for every piece of research you can find supporting one conclusion, I can find one supporting the opposite. So how do you know which is right? It comes back to academically critiquing the research to identify which is the "good" research. If both are equally as good or equally as bad, that reinforces the need for further study. If something has overwhelming evidence proving a certain conclusion, then I can say with almost certainty that it's already known by the healthcare professionals who need to know it.

I don't want to discourage you from learning and bettering your understanding of your medical problems, but I want you to be able to recognize your own limitations. We all have limitations; don't let yours get in the way of getting better care.

Keep an open mind

There is nothing more frustrating as a healthcare professional than a patient with a closed mind. It's good to know what you want in life. I applaud decisiveness. But that doesn't mean you shouldn't listen to alternatives. If you go to your appointment and you already "know" what you need, then why are you going to see a doctor in the first place?

Having an idea of what treatment is usual for your situation is a good thing, but there may be reasons an alternate course is needed. You should be open to this, and be prepared to talk about it and discuss it. You know, like an adult. If a toddler came to you demanding candy ten minutes before you were about to serve dinner, what would you say? Would the child get what he or she wanted? Of course not. When you approach your appointment in the same way the toddler approached his or her situation, you set yourself up for the same result. It's not wise to put your doctor on the defensive. Your doctor is there to help you and is putting your needs first. Truly. So don't make your doctor feel like she is superfluous or a means to an end. If you do, you're less likely to leave your appointment happy with your treatment plan, which means you probably won't stick to it, either, and that helps no one. I'm not saying you should blindly listen to your doctor and accept her word as gospel. Far from it. But in order to make an informed decision about your treatment plan, you need to know about the alternatives. Have an open mind when you go to your doctor's appointment, and you may be surprised at just how much of a difference it makes.

Keeping track yourself

If you have a chronic illness, you will have something that needs to be monitored. Whether it's pain, blood sugar, bowel movements, or your mood, something will need to be managed. Keeping a diary of that something helps you both. The doctor's happy because she can quickly see any patterns that may need investigating. It cuts down on the amount of questions she needs to ask you, which saves time. It also gives her a picture of progress or regress without bias. As a human being, I have bias. It's not always conscious, but when my own pain is worse over a period of time, my perception of my pain control and disease skews a little. It seems worse. The opposite is also true—when I have a prolonged period of mild pain, I feel like "I've got this." Your own mindset on any particular day, especially with regard to pain, will influence your doctor's appointment and the answers you give. It is important that you realize this and that you be mindful of it when you're sitting with the doctor. A diary will help you get a clear perspective of your own condition, too. It reminds you on bad days that you have had, and will continue to have, good days. On your good days, it will remind you to keep to your treatment plan because it's working. It will also remind you to be prepared for when the next bad day comes, because, unfortunately, there will likely be another bad day at some point. It happens to the best of us.

Think long-term

Chronic illness by definition is long-term, which

means management will be long and slow. I know this is kind of obvious, but it is important to keep in mind when you set your appointment goals, which we will do later. Don't get upset with your doctor for not addressing all of your issues. Your doctor will have in her head a list of priorities, which will be based on your discussion. Some things will just have to wait— not only because of time constraints, but sometimes because the smaller problems, which may feel like big problems to you, may resolve or get better by tackling the other issues first. One thing I have found is that doctors do not always communicate this to patients very well, and they should.

Be prepared for your appointment

We've mentioned that doctors want to know you are taking your health, and its care, seriously. Showing you have planned for the appointment helps achieve this. Your care shouldn't be one-sided; it should involve give and take. You and your doctor working together as a team. Laying some groundwork shows you are willing to do your part, and not rely on the doctor to "fix" you.

So how do you plan for an appointment? I'm glad you asked, because that leads us into the next chapter, "Planning."

CHAPTER FOUR

Planning

Why plan?

Although the premise of this book is to make your appointments more productive, which will ultimately lead to better care, it is not the only reason you should concentrate your efforts on planning. In fact, depending on your own situation, it may not even be the number one reason.

Going to a doctor's appointment, for some, is anxiety-inducing, especially if it's with a doctor you haven't seen before. This isn't necessarily a bad thing, because it shows you care. As an underlying theme, showing you care should be one of the reasons you plan. Nobody gets anxious for something they don't care about. If a doctor sees you're anxious, he knows this is very important to you, and that's a good thing.

If you're someone who gets anxious at appointments, you won't need me to explain the crippling effect it can have. Leaving an appointment feeling like you achieved nothing is frustrating, at best. I've had that feeling before, too. Couldn't say I care to repeat it.

Planning out your appointment will help achieve all these things. It will help you reduce your anxiety and demonstrate that you care about your health and how it's managed, and it will help you be more efficient with your time. There really is no reason not to plan.

Setting long- and short-term goals

Deciding on your short- and long-term goals will help you plan your whole appointment. Sharing these goals with your doctor will inform him about what's important to you right now, helping you achieve your goals. This will only happen if your goals are achievable. It can be easy to dream up the perfect scenario where your condition is gone, or where you're completely pain-free every day. These goals sound good but often are unrealistic. You are better served to aim for achievable goals. Meeting a goal will give you a sense of achievement and a confidence boost, helping you feel more in control of your disease.

I always feel it's better to have more than one goal at a time. Two, to be precise: one short-term goal and one long-term. By setting two goals, I know I can meet several short-term goals in the time it takes to meet my long-term goal. This helps me stay focused on always moving forward and helps me feel more in control of my illness. You may not be able to set two goals if your condition is stable or in remission, but as long as you have at least one goal, you'll be able to plan your appointment with a specific purpose in mind. Setting too many goals at once will, of course, make your objectives confusing for you and your doctor, because you won't be able to tackle them all at once.

How to set your goals

There are a few important things to keep in mind when setting your goals. Let's go over them quickly, so you can get started and write down your goals.

I hope you are familiar already with the goal-setting term SMART. I first came across the term in high school, and it is still relevant. In fact, it still seems to be a standard framework by which goals are set. A simple Google (or Bing) search for "goal setting" will yield countless references to the five-step process. So let's get to it:

S is for specific—A specific goal could be: reduce my blood pressure to 140/80. Or reduce my daily pain score from 6/10 to 3/10. Having a specific goal will help you plan appropriately. Vague goals leave the door open for interpretation by your doctor, which means he or she might not have the same outcome in mind as you. If you set the vague goal of reducing your pain, your doctor may consider it a success if your pain is reduced from 6/10 to 5/10. Except it's not. Your expectation was 3/10. Be specific and don't leave your goals open to interpretation.

M is for measurable—This is obvious, right? It can go hand in hand with "specific." Once you put a number on something, you've made it both measurable and specific. It also means that targets that are not measurable often are harder to achieve, because they are harder to define. In reality, almost anything can be measured but in healthcare there will always be symptoms that can be difficult to measure but will still require treatment. If you don't think you can measure your problem, Google (or Bing) it with the word "scale" or "score" after it. You'll be amazed to find the ways in which some things are measured.

A is for achievable—This goes back to the point I made earlier. If it's not achievable, you are not helping yourself. Start with what can be changed. Then, once there's nothing left, shoot for the stars.

R is for relevant—Have different goals for each specialist you see. Don't go to your dermatologist and tell him or her about your goal to reduce your cholesterol. Likewise, don't expect your cardiologist to help you with that rash. They may be perfectly good goals, but set different ones with each specialist. Your primary care doctor or general practitioner (GP) is the only exception to this. He needs to know it all.

T is for time-bound—Have you ever heard of Parkinson's Law? It explains, "Work expands so as to fill the time available for its completion."[3] If you don't set yourself a deadline, you run the risk of never achieving your goals. Setting a time frame will also help you to prioritize your goals if you have several. Is your next doctor's appointment in three months' time? That's a good time frame for a lot of short-term goals. If it's a long-term goal, maybe one year from now is better. You get the idea.

Addressing your barriers

Your barriers need to be broken down before you can start to plan your appointments. You can do all the prep in the world, but if you don't address your barrier(s), then it is unlikely your appointments will be productive.

Go back to what we did earlier when we identified your barrier(s). Did you write one down? I hope so. If not, go back and do it now.

With that done, we need to figure out how to overcome it. Physical barriers are normally the easiest to solve. Personal barriers are normally the hardest, because they require a change to your habits or mindset.

Your barrier(s) are unique to you. I cannot tell you how to break your barrier(s) down unless I know what they are first. Identifying your barrier(s) is half the battle. Once you've done that, breaking them down becomes easier. Here are a few examples to help you get started:

Too shy to talk

I'm not a shy person these days, but I used to be. I've found that shyness often comes from lack of confidence. That was the case for me. If this describes you, then you may want to work on building your confidence so you can speak up. This won't come easily, but it is certainly achievable. You're not alone. In fact, in my experience, it is quite a common barrier. So much so, I decided to write a whole section on it later in this book. Taking steps to build your confidence will have a significant impact on your care. There are two experts in the room when it comes to your health—your doctor and you. Sometimes both sides forget that.

"They don't understand what I want"

Do you feel like your doctor may have different goals from yours? This is another common barrier. The reason for this will vary from person to person. First, do you know what you want? This might seem like a silly question, but is it? Do you honestly know what you want? Did you set a goal? If you did, then tell your doctor. Be blunt, if needed. Make sure you're both on the same page. Being clear with your doctor about your expectations will help him understand your feelings. Your doctor should also do the same, of course. If you have been clear about your expectations, but you don't know where your doctor stands, then you need to be assertive and ask him to give that information freely.

"I never know where I need to go, and I can't walk very far"

Being forced to do something you are unable to do—such as walk a long way—will certainly make you anxious. Sensible planning often will solve this problem, but it will only work if you can admit you need help. Your barrier might not be as straightforward as you think. If you're trying to do everything yourself, even if you can't, then you will not break down your barrier. Struggling to admit to yourself, and to others, that you need help might be the actual barrier. Logistical barriers are easily overcome on their own. You can call the reception desk and ask for directions to the clinic. They will also be able to tell you if there are elevators and disabled-accessible facilities. They might be able to provide you with a wheelchair and take you to your appointment on arrival. Each hospital or clinic is different, but this information is freely available if you ask. If you let your stubbornness get in the way of receiving help, then you will never break down your true barrier.

Considering other specialists' input

It's not uncommon to see more than one specialist.

Keeping up with several doctors can be exhausting, but for some people it's a necessary evil. The communication among your doctors can vary widely. It can be dismal, or it can be encouraging. I have spoken to many people who have had experiences on both ends of the spectrum, and many in between. Different healthcare providers do things differently and, unfortunately, you're the one who gets stuck in the middle making sure they all play nicely together.

The plans of one doctor can have profound impact on the plans of another. I hope that's obvious, but it's easy sometimes to forget. We see this doctor for this problem and that doctor for that problem. By compartmentalizing your care this way, you may very easily assume everything has defined borders, but usually they overlap. Sometimes that's difficult to see with the structure of healthcare we have these days. This happens all over the world, and not just in the United States and United Kingdom.

If your doctors talk to each other, through whatever medium, then consider your job half-done. If they don't, for whatever reason (maybe you started seeing a new doctor), then your first job is to open the lines of communication. So take the contact details of the other specialists you see with you to your appointments. Also, write down, as briefly as possible, the current plan of action and what future goals you and your specialist(s) have. Knowing these could have a dramatic effect on what treatments your doctor offers you, as well as what goals you set together. It's always better for your doctors to know these early on.

The hard part of discussing another specialist's input at your doctor's appointment is knowing what is relevant. My advice is to keep it simple. Summarize each doctor's action plan and future goals. Let your other doctor know this at your appointment. This opens the door, and it's then up to your doctor to walk through it. If your doctor needs to know more, he will ask. Just summarizing it in this way often will be enough, so don't be upset or disappointed if your doctor doesn't ask for more detail. Just be ready in case he does.

Outstanding issues

By now you should expect that if you have multiple problems, it is unlikely they will all be addressed in one short appointment, and that's okay. But it's important not to forget them entirely. It's good to keep an ongoing record of them, with some sort of note as to when they were addressed last and how.

You may find that you keep adding to this list and

that some problems keep getting ignored. While it is important to prioritize your issues, and frankly I advise it, it is also important not to leave any neglected without an answer. So, it may well be time to mention it at your next appointment, even if the answer is, "We'll deal with that once X is dealt with." Now, although you haven't taken any steps to solve that issue and it's still on your list, at least you have an answer.

It is also important to ensure that any issue you raise, even if it's not being addressed at this time, is noted or mentioned in your appointment summary/medical notes by the doctor. The old adage, "If it's not written down it didn't happen," applies. Your doctor won't remember that it was mentioned or discussed. If it's in your notes, then even if he doesn't remember, he can see it was discussed and will be more inclined to revisit it on your next appointment without you having to bring it up again.

The take-away advice is: Make a list of all your issues. Cross them off when dealt with; mark them when discussed or pending. Don't let anything be forgotten.

Documentation

Paperwork, paperwork, paperwork. If there's one thing healthcare loves, it's damn paperwork. It is, of course, a necessary evil. Many doctors may have switched to electronic paperwork, which does save time, but it is still considered a time sink. Regardless of which method your doctor uses, the ability to communicate effectively with you and with other healthcare professionals is paramount to your care and safety.

As the patient, you need to manage your own share of the administrative load. Some people find this easy and some don't, but in either case being organized with your documentation is key to helping you have a productive doctor's appointment. Having everything ready for the doctor saves time. It also shows the doctor that you are responsible and that you care about your health and its management (there's that theme again).

More importantly, for some, being organized will help reduce anxiety and stress before the appointment. I'm sure we all at some point have forgotten to take something basic to an appointment. I know I have. Finding out you've forgotten an important letter or test result can bring on stress or anxiety. At the very least, it's annoying, and it starts you off on the wrong foot, so let's get it right from the start. The following sections are the key areas to consider when preparing your documents.

The obvious

I shouldn't need to remind you of the following things, but I will, as people do forget them. They don't forget these documents because they didn't think to bring them, but instead, because they failed to create any workable organizational system for themselves. Don't be that person. Get a folder specifically for your health documents. Then you only have one thing to remember, instead of trying to remember each individual document. I'm a fan of color-coded page dividers, too. They help separate my documents by type, with a different one for each doctor. And I make sure my documents are in order! My most recent are on the top, going backwards in time to my earliest appointments. Over the years, you'll find you run out of room. There's nothing wrong with taking some old documents out and archiving them. Just maintain the order if you do, keeping at least the past year's papers, if not two to three years' worth, in your current folder.

1. **Insurance card**

This depends on which country you reside in, of course, but make sure you don't get stuck with a hefty bill unnecessarily, because you forgot your insurance card. It's also a good idea to know ahead of time what medicines your insurance covers, as well as knowing your copays. Read your insurance documents to make sure you are informed before your appointment. It is hard to know, especially with a new doctor, what treatments he may offer, so this can be tricky, but knowing the common treatment options for your case will help you research what is and is not covered. This may impact your decisions later. There are few things more frustrating than deciding on a treatment, then realizing it is not covered by your insurance, leaving you to decide whether to pursue an alternate treatment (if there is one) or to pay the whole cost of the treatment. It's not a decision I would want anyone to make.

2. ID

This, again, is something that is mostly only for the United States, because the insurance companies want to know it's actually you seeing the doctor and making the claim. But on some rare occasions you need this in the United Kingdom. Most people usually carry some form of ID on them anyway, as they often have their driver's license on their person. If you don't drive, make sure you have an alternate form of ID.

3. Up-to-date contact details

When I was a practicing nurse, there were far too many times when I tried to call patients, only to realize their contact numbers were outdated. So frustrating! It's the simplest thing to correct, but it can cause the most difficult problems. After all, I'm not calling to chat—I'm calling for a reason. Any half-decent reception team will ask you if your details have changed. But that doesn't always happen, no matter on which side of the pond you live. If you've recently moved or got a new phone number, make sure you update your information with your doctors. For those in the United States, this means updating it with your insurance provider, too. If you're in the United Kingdom, then change it with each hospital you visit, as well as with your GP. If it is changed on one system, don't assume it is changed on all, because they *do not* sync together. The same can apply for those in the United States. Occasionally, through human or computer error, when you do update your details, it doesn't save, so make sure to check the next time you go. This may seem like I'm putting a lot of importance on something minor, but I'm doing it for a reason. If your medical team cannot contact you and there is something wrong, it can have serious implications for your health. Sometimes things are time-sensitive and need to be dealt with immediately. Check, double-check, and check again.

Doctor's letters or appointment summaries

The United Kingdom and United States have very different systems for managing and recording health records. In both cases, you will have a record, which will be needed by a new doctor or service provider. If you live outside of these regions, you still will need to take records with you. As for the specifics, I can't help you. But the takeaway message is: Take your records with you to new appointments. So let's break it down by region:

United Kingdom—Your specialist will write a letter to your GP explaining your appointment and treatments prescribed. You should get a copy mailed to you automatically. If you do not receive a copy, I would not recommend asking your GP for one. This is a slow process, and he may not have it yet, either. It takes time to process these letters, and that is a big downside to using a paper system (though that is slowly changing). What you should do is contact your doctor's secretary, who is otherwise known as the "gatekeeper" (and for good reason). A good secretary is a joyous thing—he solves problems and appears to make light work of difficult tasks. A stressed and overworked one will often leave you wanting to pull out your hair. Be prepared for the latter. If you have a previous letter from that doctor, the phone number will be on the letter. Note: You cannot call the doctor directly in the NHS—you have to go through the secretary. If it was a first appointment, call the hospital's switchboard and ask to be put through to your doctor's secretary. There's a good chance he won't pick up. Having shared an office with several secretaries, I can tell you with absolute authority that their phones ring ALL day long. And I mean, literally, they don't stop. It's like being in a call center. If they answered every call, they would never get anything else done, so be prepared to leave a voice mail. Make sure you have your details ready so you can leave a clear and concise message. You will need your name, your date of birth, your hospital number, and a contact phone number in case they need to call you back.

If you're seeing a new doctor or specialist, you may find other specialists' input is important. So if you see other doctors, take their letters with you, too. When you see a GP, you won't have a letter. It would be rather a waste if he wrote a letter to himself. But he can provide a health summary, which will list your current and previous medical problems and your medications. This summary is normally sent by your GP, along with the referral, to the new specialist, but it's good to know how to get a copy if you need to.

United States—Depending on your state and healthcare provider, this may vary slightly. America is ahead of the United Kingdom when it comes to digital records. This is mostly a good thing. It means you can access them online at your own leisure, in most cases. This cuts out the need to make phone calls, etc., should you need to obtain copies of your records. But not everyone is tech-savvy, nor does everyone have easy access to the internet. This poses a problem for those people who often need paper copies the most. In this instance, I would advise that at the end of each appointment, you ask for a copy of your appointment summary. In my experience, the staff are always happy to oblige. Failing this, you should be able to call the clinic or hospital directly for a copy. This won't be the easiest or the quickest method by far, but it shouldn't be too much of a headache. Just make sure, if you do call, to have your insurance details, such as your medical record/patient number, ready, along with the date of the appointment for which you wish to get the record.

Areas of concern

I like lists. I'm not ashamed to admit it. Lists are cool. They leave me satisfied when I tick things off. Are you one of those kinds of people, too? It's okay if not; I won't judge. But now we get to write one. Yay!

When you have one or more chronic illnesses, you always have more than one problem to deal with. As we've already mentioned, you aren't going to get all your areas of concern addressed in one 10-to-15-minute appointment, so you need to prioritize your problems and deal with what you consider the most important first. The easiest way is to write a regular, old-fashioned list. Brainstorm all your problems or needs that need to be addressed, and write them down as you go. Then you can number the problems from most to least important and reorder your list. Easy, right? Good.

You may be wondering: How to know what's the most important? Well, that's really up to you. You are an individual with your own personal needs and concerns, so the right answer is what you say it is. You may find as you brainstorm and write your list that it orders itself. The most important issues to you will most likely come to mind first and be first on your list.

It's important to keep in mind that the most pressing concerns for you may not be the most pressing for your doctor. We touched on this earlier. That's okay, as you are looking at your issues from different perspectives. But you both need to communicate this to each other. Without that communication, you will head on different paths. The most successful path is the one you are both on. So now take your list, and next to each concern write the "why." Why is it important to you? What impact is it having on your life? Do this for each item on your list. Qualify it, and make sure it deserves to be on your list. If you can't think of a reason for it to be on your list, then maybe it doesn't need to be there. That's your call, but it's worth considering. Having the "why" will help you express your areas of concern to your doctor. It will help convey the sense of importance you place on it, helping the doctor understand you and your problems a little better.

Just a quick final note. This list should be dynamic. Items should be added, taken away and reordered as appropriate. Things change in our social and economic lifestyles, and undoubtedly this will have an impact on your priorities in life. Don't be afraid to bump things down on the list if they become not as important to you. Just remember, if you add new items to the list, make sure you add the "why," too.

Questions to ask

Before any doctor's appointment, you are going to have questions, regardless of the problem and how long you've had it. Even someone who has been managing a chronic illness for twenty years has questions, because our health is rarely static. Something is always changing for better or for worse.

Therefore, it is key that these questions are answered, along with any new ones that crop up during the appointment. The best and most obvious way of getting this done is to list your questions beforehand and take them with you. You can ask these questions at the most appropriate point during your appointment. When that is depends solely on what your questions are, so you'll have to figure that one out yourself. In any case, you will need to review the questions and answers at the end of the appointment to make sure that you have a satisfactory answer, or at least know where to go to get that answer. If you have unanswered questions from your last appointment, I'd suggest starting your appointment with those, unless they are unrelated to the reason for the current visit.

The questions you have for your doctor are very personal to you, but below I have listed a few general questions that you might need to consider or add to your list:

<u>Before an appointment</u>

- What is causing my problem?

- Is there more than one condition that could cause it?

- Does my insurance cover my tests and treatment options?

During an appointment

- What are the tests for?

- When will I get the results? (And whom do you contact if you don't get the results?)

- What are my treatment options?

- What will happen if we do nothing?

- Are there any side effects? How common are they?

- How effective is this treatment? What should I expect?

- How long is the treatment?

- Is there anything I should not do/eat while on this treatment?

- Does it adversely interact with any of my current

medications?

- What changes can I make in my lifestyle to make a difference?

<u>Ending an appointment</u>

- Is there any written information I can take home on this?

- Is there an online/physical support group or charity for this condition? (Very important if you've been newly diagnosed with a chronic condition.)

- Do I need to contact you if things get worse? If so, how? (email, phone, etc.)

- Do I need to come back again? When is my next appointment?

Medication list

If you haven't changed any of your medication for years, and you are seeing the same doctor, this isn't so important. Otherwise, I would recommend you keep a copy of your medication list with you when you visit any of your doctors. They may already be on the doctor's computer, and that's great, but what isn't there is why was there a change, or why you stopped taking a particular medication. This is as important as the list itself. I would suggest you keep a list of your medications and next to them put a start date, end date, and reason for stopping. Sometimes it's as important to know what medications you've tried in the past when dealing with a difficult-to-manage problem (pain, for instance) than it is to know what you're taking now. An example of a medication list is in the "Resources" section of this book.

Please also be meticulous and write down all of what you take, not just those medications that are prescribed. Don't assume that because it was bought over the counter, or it's a natural or herbal remedy, that it isn't important. Some of these can have quite serious side effects that are not necessarily advertised, which will affect your care. We discussed some of these earlier in the "What doctors expect from you" section. So please write down every supplement and homeopathic medication you're taking. Include any cold and flu remedies, too. Absolutely everything. If this list is extensive, consider organizing it to keep the current medications at the top of the list and stopped ones toward the bottom for easy reading. You could also use color to help organize them, or use the strikethrough function (if using an Excel or Word document). However you decide to present it, make it easily readable for all.

Symptom history

This is not to be confused with the previous section, "Areas of concern." It can be easy for these to overlap, and if they do, that's fine. In our previous list we needed to know the "why," where instead here we need to know a lot more detail.

I've created a symptom history sheet you can download and use to help you follow along. It can be found by going to the "Resources" section of this book. You are, of course, free to make your own version should the presentation of mine not appeal to you, or you can adjust my version to meet your own preferences.

We could just make a list, as we did in the previous section. Boy, do I love lists. But that wouldn't suffice in this case. We need more detail. One of the benefits of doing all this now is that it will save time in your appointment, because you can just read off the sheet or show it to the doctor to read. There is no wasted time thinking about a question before you answer, then realizing you forgot something or got your dates wrong. One of the other benefits, just like with our "Areas of concern" list, is that it helps you organize your thoughts and give each item on the sheet some form of priority or importance. This will help you down the road.

As for what to add to this list, you can include any symptoms—physical, mental, or otherwise. Generally, it's a good idea to note more than just the physical. This list also is for all your symptoms, not just ones related to a specific illness you have. Write it all down.

Again, this history sheet is meant to be dynamic. It will change after each appointment and as each symptom has been attended to. You can print this sheet and fill it in by hand if you wish, but I would recommend filling it in on your computer and printing it off when you need to (assuming you have the facilities to do so). This will save you from rewriting the list now and then as things get added and removed. It's a task that is much easier on a computer.

For this list, you are going to have seven sections, as follows:

Symptom—Keep it simple. The details are going to follow in the following sections. One to three words should suffice in most cases. For example, "heartburn" or "lower back pain."

Duration & frequency—How often do you get it?

Daily? Weekly? Or is it constant? How long does it last when you do have it? You get the idea.

Cause—Now comes the detail. What causes it? You may not know. And that's cool. Leave it blank until the day comes when you find out. If you do know, write it down. For example, "after I eat" or "when I sit down."

Relief—So we know what causes it, but now the doctor will want to know what helps relieve it. What do you do to help? Take a medication? Stretch? Change position? Drink a glass of milk? Whatever "works" (in the loose sense of the word) should be noted in this section. Also, note if the symptom goes away completely or not. Maybe it just "takes the edge off."

Start date—This is hopefully self-explanatory. Note when it first appeared. Simple.

End date—Fill this section in when one of the following happens. Note the date if the symptom goes away because of an intervention, such as if a new medication is taken to treat it. Sometimes things just go away of their own accord, but it's still something that should be recorded. After all, it could come back again in the future.

Action taken—A simple sentence detailing the steps taken to help relieve or reduce the symptom. For example, "medication prescribed" or "stopped eating fried food."

I hope this helps you get a handle on your symptoms. As you can see, there potentially is a lot of information needed by the doctor for each symptom. Having it recorded in detail in a fairly easy-to-read format makes life easier for both you and your doctor, saving you a whole bunch of time in your appointment.

Disease-specific documents

The last thing you should consider when collating your documents is anything that is specific to your disease that will be helpful during the appointment. Most long-term diseases require you to monitor some aspect of your health, such as blood pressure or blood sugar. But it's not always something you can prepare for. For example, there's nothing you can do prior to your appointment if you're getting a standard blood test. Others, however, can be. Let's use mine as an example.

For my disease, ankylosing spondylitis, there is a score which is referred to as a BASDAI score (Bath Ankylosing Spondylitis Disease Activity Index)[4].

This is a one-page sheet of paper with six questions that ask me to rate, on a scale of 0 to 10, my symptoms, such as pain and stiffness. The doctor would hand me a copy of it and ask me on the spot to fill it out. Can you see where this going? Yeah, what a waste of time. Not only did it take time to fill out, but I felt pressured and rushed to do it quickly. It is not something you should rush. It is something you should think about carefully, even if just to be consistent. I always hated filling it out in front of the doctor. It was never easy for me to think of the answers quickly, especially when I was thinking back over the whole week, as in one question, so it always made me a little anxious. After far too long, it finally occurred to me. Why can't I do this in my own time before the appointment? I looked online and found a PDF version of the BASDAI score. Excellent. So before my next appointment, I printed it off and filled it in. I made sure to put my name, my medical record number, and the date at the top (this is very important). My doctor didn't mind I filled it out previously, because I had dated it. In fact, I made time to do it that same day before my appointment. Not only did I save time, but it helped me feel less rushed in my appointment.

Do you have something similar that you do each time that is specific to your disease? Then do what I did. Do the work beforehand and have it ready to present to your doctor. Make sure that any paper documentation you hand to the doctor has your name and medical record / hospital number on it, and, most importantly, the date it was filled out. If you don't include all of those, then your doctor will do it, and that takes time. He will be more thankful if you hand him a completed document that needs nothing from him other than the reading of it. Doctors hate paperwork, so don't make them fill out anything you've missed.

Managing multiple appointments

If you have a chronic illness, the one thing you can guarantee is that you'll have lots of doctors' appointments. You may even feel like it's your second home (been there, done that).

You also will likely see more than one doctor, and may even have enough to fill a basketball team. Keeping track of them all will be a challenge, even for the least forgetful of us.

There are many systems you can use to keep track, and at the end of the day it'll be your personal preference, but there are a few things you will need to consider in each case. I have made a resource sheet for you to download should managing your appointments be something you struggle with, or is something you are new to. Once again, you can find it at in the "Resources" section.

Not only will a good system prevent you from missing an appointment, which is obviously key to actually getting any care, but it also will help you with your planning and preparation for those appointments. For instance, having the dates of your future appointments on hand might be useful for one of your other doctors, because he may wish to follow up and discuss something with your other doctors (not you) following your visit.

Date and time

Okay, Captain Obvious strikes again! Have you ever arranged a doctor's appointment, only to realize later you had something else planned and had to move your appointment? Yep, I've been there, too. It happens to the best of us. At least that's what I tell myself.

Whatever system you have, make sure you can easily cross-check your calendar to make sure you do not double-book. Moving your appointment later may mean your three-month check turns into four months, or, worse, six months. ~~Measure twice, cut~~

~~once~~. Check twice, arrange once.

Who is it with?

Don't assume, especially if your doctor is part of a team. Although your next appointment may be with a specialist, say a rheumatologist, is it the same doctor, or just another rheumatologist from the same team or building? Maybe your doctor is on vacation, so you get to see whoever is covering. This makes a huge difference in terms of how you approach your preparation for the appointment.

Seeing someone other than your usual doctor isn't always bad, so don't assume that it will be. For proof, see my story at the back of the book. My patient journey would look remarkably different (in a negative way) if it wasn't for a stand-in doctor.

Where is it?

Again, always double-check. Maybe that day they are repainting the halls, so your appointment is on a different floor. And don't be the person who turns up to the correct department, but at the wrong hospital or offices. It happens, and to an extent, it's understandable, but it almost always could have been avoided with proper preparation.

Did you arrange your follow-up appointment?

After your appointment, you most likely will need to go back if you've seen a specialist, whether it's in days, weeks, or months. Sometimes you may not be able to arrange your next appointment right away, depending on how your healthcare provider does its scheduling. It's important to document whether you still need to arrange a follow-up appointment. It's easy to forget, and then, yet again, your three-month follow-up turned into a six month follow-up. I've yet to come across a service that reminds you to book an appointment if you haven't done so already. If you know of one, I'd love to hear about it. Send me an email.

Approaching a first appointment

The manner in which you approach an appointment with a doctor you're seeing for the first time is different from that of a follow-up. For your first appointment, the doctor will be focused on your medical history and what led you to this point in time. It sounds obvious, but it does change how you approach your planning.

You should also expect the appointment to be

repetitive in that you'll be asked questions and have tests repeated that you may have had recently. There is good reason for this, so don't be annoyed at your doctor for "wasting time." Trust me, he wouldn't do it if he didn't need to. Physical exams especially are almost always repeated, particularly if you're seeing a specialist.

From the doctor's perspective, getting a solid baseline of tests to work from is key to managing your health, as is getting an accurate medical history. This is even more the case if you're seeing a specialist, because specialists want to know what led you to being referred to them. So you will need to make sure that you are dressed appropriately for the tests and exams needed. You also will need to make sure that your documentation is up-to-date and organized. You will need easy access to different papers at certain points—complete medication lists, vaccination history, symptoms list, past blood test results (if you have access to them), and a summary of your other medical problems are the bare minimum of what you need to take with you.

When it comes to your goals, you should concentrate on communicating your short-term goals at the first appointment, and then introduce your long-term goals at the second appointment (unless you're asked otherwise by the doctor—in which case, great! He's a keeper). I feel this is a good idea because, firstly, you won't have much time because you've spent most of your appointment getting your baselines, and secondly, you don't want to start overwhelming your doctor with issues at the start. By limiting what you want to achieve (in the first appointment only), you're letting him know what is important to you right now, which gives a sense of priority to your short-term goal. If you start trying to solve everything at once, then you start diminishing the importance of the goals that are most important to you.

Consider this first appointment the same as laying the foundation for your house. Without a good foundation, even the prettiest and well-thought-out house will tumble. A good foundation is easier to build on, just as a good first impression makes it easier to build a good working relationship with your doctor. That's not to say you can't develop a good relationship out of a bad one. It is possible, but it will take a lot more time, and a lot more give-and-take, to achieve it.

Approaching a follow-up appointment

When you see a doctor for a follow-up appointment, whether for the second or for the hundredth time, the focus of your planning should be different from that of a first appointment. While the focus of a first appointment is mostly historic, the focus of subsequent appointments should be looking forward.

Have you noticed that I haven't mentioned the now? What about looking at what's happening right now? Now is temporary and short-sighted. Of course it needs to be addressed, but that can be done at the current appointment, regardless of whether it's a new appointment or follow-up. The issue with "now" is that it changes. Each appointment has its own "now." Focusing on that is often counterproductive. Let's use a common example, which is somewhat personal, to explain what I mean:

Scenario:

I attend my follow-up appointment for my chronic illness on time and prepared. My daily pain levels are increasing slowly, to the point that I'm in rather a lot of pain. The doctor asks me how I'm doing, and I explain the pain. We talk options to control my pain. We have a healthy discussion. I'm informed and know all the side effects. We come to a decision on the best medication to try to help me relieve my pain. I walk away from the appointment satisfied that I was listened to. I feel informed and included in the treatment of my problem.

This is good, right? I came away satisfied. I was listened to. We worked together to come up with the best plan of action for me. So what is the problem with this very common scenario?

The problem is, it is only looking at the "now". Even if my medication works, I may still be in pain. Maybe it doesn't work well enough, or maybe I experienced side effects. One of my mottos in life is, "Always have a Plan B." And if you can, have a Plan C too. There are two things missing from the scenario. The first being, there was no Plan B. What happens if the medication doesn't work? Do I call or email him? Do I just stop the medication? Is there an alternative medication to try if the primary one fails? I won't see my doctor again for three months. That's a long time to be in pain.

The second problem with this scenario is more concerning. The question "why" is absent. Why am I in pain? It may be obvious, especially if my pain is related to my chronic illness, but what's being done about it long-term? What are we—the doctor and I—

going to do to prevent it happening again? We never discussed how we could address the cause of the problem. We just focused on the symptom. It's easy for both parties to concentrate on the "now," especially when you both feel like you are making a difference. But it's not productive in the long term.

I should state at this point that if you have a condition that flares up, and you have an extra appointment to deal with the flare-up, you should definitely be focusing on the "now". But for all other appointments, the focus should always be looking forward.

We've talked about long-term goals already. Make sure they aren't neglected for the "now." So, if need be, interrupt the flow of the appointment and change its focus to what you both can do to help long-term. Even if your long-term goal is very long-term (for instance, years), it still should be mentioned briefly at each follow-up appointment to make sure you're still on track and it is still a relevant and appropriate goal. Your heath will change over time; it's important that your goals change with them.

One way you can help direct your focus for the appointment is through reflection. There is a whole chapter on reflective accounts later in this book, so you'll get to learn how to apply it later, but your reflection after your previous appointment will help highlight what you need to include in your planning of this appointment. Don't worry, it'll all become clear later. For now, just remember to revise your previous reflective account before your current appointment.

We've also talked about addressing your barriers. You may also find that as time goes on new barriers appear. This is another reason to revisit your previous reflection, which will help you identify any new issues that are stopping you from getting the quality of care you deserve. Be sure to include those in your planning of your follow-up appointment.

We compared a first doctor appointment to laying the foundation of a house. That would make the follow-up appointments the building of the house. Once a house is built, does it always stay the same? Not usually. We redecorate, remodel, and renovate. The same is true with your doctor's appointments. Be afraid of the status quo. Staying the same may well be appealing, especially if you've been going backward for so long, but you should always aim to go forward. If the best you achieve is the status quo, that's fine. Just don't make that your aim.

Do you use a washing machine to clean your clothes? Or do you go scrub them in the river? Both methods work, but sometimes new things come along that are just better. The same is true for medical treatments. New treatments are constantly becoming available. Maybe there's a better one for you. Don't be scared of change. Be excited by it and embrace it.

CHAPTER FIVE

Effective Communication

Why bother?

Sometimes the thing that holds us back the most isn't our planning or our mindset, but instead our ability to execute our plans and desires. Not everyone is a good communicator. That applies to both sides of the desk. And that's okay. Not everyone can be, nor should it be expected. We are individuals with our own strengths and weaknesses. As long as we recognize our weaknesses, we can do something about them.

We've already covered what is expected of patients and how we can prepare to make the most of our appointments. Now it's time to execute what we've learned through good communication skills.

If you're the confident type who is not afraid of speaking in public, then you may not find some of this chapter relevant, in which case skip over the parts you feel you don't need. If you're not that type of person, you may find this chapter helps you the most. Let's get started.

Your body language

What you don't say can be just as important as what you do say, and I'm not talking about verbally withholding information. That, of course, would be bad, too. Instead, I'm talking about your body language and mannerisms.

We all have things we do that are not ideal. Mine is a twitch/shake in my leg, and it drives my poor wife mad. It's not something that bothers me normally, but when I visit a doctor's office I become very conscious of it. It makes me look nervous when I'm not. And if I look nervous, then I don't look confident or in control, which can be important. Sometimes the appearance of confidence is more than enough, even if you don't feel it.

Before we dig into some specifics and look at positive and negative behaviors, we should start by looking at ourselves objectively. Like I did with my problem, you need to identify any negative behavior you have and determine why it's bad. You shouldn't take this as a personal criticism. We all have some shortcoming, even the best communicators. Try and look at it objectively, as if you were trying to fix a broken car or a computer. It will become a lot easier to fix or manage once you remove the emotion. Not being a good communicator is nothing to be ashamed of. It's just another type of barrier we need to break down.

So let's look at some positive and negative body language examples. The obvious point: Do the positive ones, avoid the negative ones. The less obvious point: If you overdo or exaggerate the positive body language, it can actually appear negative, so moderation and consistency are the key.

Positive body language

Good handshake or greeting—I'm a keen believer in making a good first impression. A good handshake and a positive greeting go a long way toward forming a good impression. They also set a positive tone to start the appointment. So start practicing your handshake.

Posture—Unless your condition prevents it, you should sit upright in your chair, with your feet firmly planted on the ground. Show your doctor that you're alert and ready for the appointment. A good posture will help you achieve that.

Hands and arms—Hands are best used for talking and expressing yourself, providing they're not used to make rude gestures. Talking with your hands will put passion in your discussion without being aggressive. When you're not talking, your hands should be resting on your lap.

Eye contact—Maintaining good eye contact through your discussion shows you are engaged. Everyone knows this, but not everyone knows that eye contact also exudes confidence. Even if the look on your face is one of horror, maintaining eye contact will show you are still eager to engage, despite the negative emotions you feel. That takes confidence and determination.

Nodding—This partners well with eye contact. Showing you are listening is a good thing. You could also use a verbal confirmation, but I personally wouldn't recommend it. I prefer to use verbal confirmation as a lead-in to the discussion in which I share my views or opinion. Nodding works well when you want your doctor to continue to talk while showing her you are listening.

Humor—As long as the jokes are appropriate and avoid any potentially controversial topics, like politics, go ahead and crack some jokes. All things in moderation, mind you. A relaxing and engaging environment is what you're after. If you're uncomfortable with this method, then don't try it. Trying to force humor can often have the opposite effect.

Slow down—Time is precious. That's the whole point of this book. But speeding up your speech is not the answer. This often happens when you are nervous. Be conscious of it and slow down your speech. Things are more likely to be heard and understood, rather than missed in a barrage of information. Work on efficiency rather than speed. Don't use twenty words if five will do. Keep your points concise, and expand only when needed for clarity.

Take notes—Believe it or not, note-taking is a positive. Despite the fact that you are breaking eye contact, taking notes shows that you care enough to make sure everything discussed is remembered. Don't forget to look up occasionally, though. You don't want to be rude, and you also want to show you are listening. Remember, you're taking notes, not writing an essay—keep it short. Shorthand is a good idea, as long as you can remember what it means when you read it back.

Don't forget to smile—Sometimes smiling is hard to do when you feel unwell or are in pain. But it's important to show that you're not blaming your doctor for your problems. Smiling when appropriate helps to create a positive relationship between you, while also helping you feel—if only a little—better.

Negative body language

Yawning—This can be a hard one. Yawning isn't something you can stop yourself from doing easily, especially if you're tired. But as Yoda would say, "Try, you must." Being tired could be the reason you're at the doctor's, in which case ignore this part, but otherwise you should do your best to curb the urge to yawn. Yawning is also a sign of boredom. Don't look bored; look interested. If you are bored, maybe you should try to steer the conversation in a direction that is more helpful to you.

Getting distracted—Some of us are good at doing two things at once, but that doesn't mean you should. Focus your attention on the discussion at hand, and show that you are focused. Looking around at the posters on the walls, looking out of the window, or staring at that spider crawling across the floor might seem okay if you're still listening, but the doctor doesn't know you are still listening unless you show it.

Fidgeting—Sometimes we fidget because we're in pain or uncomfortable. That's okay, but be vocal about it and tell that to your doctor. Otherwise you come across as nervous or distracted.

Arms folded or arms behind head—Arms folded in front of your chest make you look defensive. And while putting them behind your head shows you're relaxed, it's not appropriate for a doctor's appointment. In fact, if it's your first appointment with that doctor, it may seem like you trying to assert authority by showing you're so in control you can relax about it. Being relaxed is good, but flaunting your confidence can be rude. Be mindful of that.

Impatience or checking your watch—Have a meeting to get to? Doctor running late? Unless you have another doctor's appointment, or you need to pick the kids up from school, there really is no need to check your watch. If your mind is elsewhere, it's easy for your doctor to become distracted as well. She's human, too. If you want her to concentrate on your care, you need to do so, also.

Foot tapping—Foot tapping, finger tapping, leg shaking, they're all the same. Aside from making you seem nervous, they also can be annoying as hell, and may even distract the doctor. Regardless of whether you are indeed nervous, stop it. Try to control it. Practice at home if you can.

Sitting on the edge of your chair—This gives the impression that you are getting ready to leave, or at least that you want to leave. Even if that may be the case, it's good to show you are still interested and focused on your appointment. If the chair is uncomfortable for you or causing you pain, that is another matter. If that is the case, you should communicate it to your doctor.

Touching your face—Touching your face while talking can be perceived as deceitful, especially if you cover your mouth in any way. We tend not to believe people that are hiding part of their face, so avoid being perceived as something you're not and keep your hands in your lap when not using them as you talk.

Do your dress and appearance really matter?

In short, yes.

But why? It shouldn't matter, right? There is an extensive amount of academic research based on how doctors should dress when seeing patients. Most of it is conflicting, from the samples I read, but I didn't find one single piece of research on how patients should dress. The general advice is to wear something appropriate. If you're expecting a physical exam, then make sure you're wearing something you can get on and off yourself, if possible. Things start getting tricky if you're coming from or going straight to work afterwards, and sometimes there is not much you can do about it.

Did you ever hear the phrase "dress to impress"? Usually it's aimed at job interviews. It works on the premise that first impressions matter, and looking professional, smart, and respectable will convince others that you possess those qualities yourself. Of course, we know that's not always the case. The phrase "don't judge a book by its cover" also comes to mind. So which is right? Well, the consensus is that dressing up a little—while still being practical—is preferable, mostly because it shows that you care enough about the appointment to make the effort and make a good impression. I'm not saying to wear a suit to the appointment, but shorts or sweatpants generally don't give the right impression in the beginning.

Each doctor-patient relationship is different and should be threated thusly. If you've known your doctors for a long time or have trouble dressing yourself, then maybe low-key dress such as sweatpants is the way to go, but use your judgment. It doesn't hurt to dress up a little, as long as it remains practical.

One last thing. Always, and I really can't stress this enough, always wear underwear! And that includes wearing a bra! The exception would be if you are physically unable to put one on because of your illness or condition, such as severe rheumatoid arthritis in your hands. In that case, you could wear something like a camisole to avoid any unnecessary embarrassment to either party.

Don't give the person examining you a shock. You may not be embarrassed, but she might. "But doctors don't embarrass easily, and they've seen it before," you might say. Yes, but when it is unexpected and unnecessary, then it can embarrass some. So unless you've been given specific orders to not do so, wear underwear, always!

What not to say, and how you can say it better

In order to improve your communication with your doctor, and thus your relationship, you need to look at your speech and not just your body language. You may be disappointed when I say this, but there are no magic words or phrases you can memorize to make things happen. It just doesn't work that way. When I first started on my journey, I thought such phrases might exist, so I looked for them, and I asked my medical colleagues. I found nothing. So if they do exist, they are the best-kept secret since the location of the Holy Grail.

I want to start by reemphasizing a point I made earlier—always tell the truth. If you start trying to bend the truth to get the care you want, you may do yourself more harm in the long run. It also does nothing to build a trusting relationship, and when it comes to chronic illness and health, you want to make sure you are building a long-term relationship with your doctor, because your health is long-term.

So now that that's out of the way, let's get into some things you definitely should not say, even if they are true. Please don't just read the headline and skip over these sections. I will be covering what you should say instead in each case. Let's get to it.

1. Bragging about firing other doctors

At no point—ever—is bragging about firing your old doctor a good thing. There is not one instance where it is even remotely helpful. Now if you say, "I'm here today for a second opinion," that's fine. It's an informative and honest sentence. It is not negative, abusive, or derogatory, like "firing" someone.

She may have been the worst doctor in the world (statistically unlikely) and may have deserved to be "fired." But when you sit on the other side of the desk and hear someone brag about firing another doctor, your first thought is, "Why?" And not "why did you," but "why are you telling me?" The natural assumption, wrongly or rightly, is that you (the bragging patient) are trying to assert some form of dominance by showing how the doctor's fate will be the same should she displease you. We humans are mammals, and just like many other Mammalia, when one starts sticking out her chest and parading around, so does the other. And before you know it, like a pair of stags, you're locking horns.

Hopefully you get the point. It's not conducive to a healthy doctor-patient relationship. The same is also true for the next point.

2. Speaking poorly about other physicians

This is almost identical to "bragging about firing other doctors." The points for that also apply here, but I'd also like to mention tone and consistency. If you find yourself on more than one occasion making a flippant or blatantly negative comment about another doctor, while at the time it could be shrugged off, over time these repetitive comments do damage. They gnaw away at your relationship like a woodworm to your beams, and before you know it, the ceiling comes crashing down. Don't be a woodworm. Instead, only reference your other physicians when it adds value to your discussion. And if you do need to mention something because it's pertinent to your current discussion or decision, do so in a factual and neutral way. There's no need to be positive about something that is by nature negative, but there's no need to emphasize the fact, either. Stating the facts and keeping it neutral will let your doctor make her own judgments on the situation, while ensuring you maintain your own dignity and trust.

3. "Knowing" what you need

I've said this before: If you truly know what you need, why are you seeing a doctor? Your reply may likely be, "Well, because I can't prescribe medications to myself." Fair enough. So your doctor went through years of medical training and got into immense debt just so she can fill in a piece of paper at your request? Okay, maybe I'm oversimplifying and being a little aggressive, but can you see how that might make a doctor feel? Doctors genuinely want to help. If you were willing to help someone, only to be treated as nothing more than a means to an end, would you feel good about that? Unlikely. So which doctor do you think will give you the best care? The one who's being treated like a means to an end, or the one who feels involved and feels satisfaction from helping you get what you need? It's obvious, I hope. Think long-term; create a relationship that lasts so you get the best care for years to come. Don't just think about the "now."

There are times when you may well know what you need before you go to an appointment. Maybe you've been advised by a charity or organization specific to your disease, and that's great! Too many people are poorly educated about their own condition. Often, as patients, we are left to find this information out for ourselves. This is not acceptable to me, but that's for another day. So knowing what you want and demanding what you want are two different things. Don't be demanding. Be willing to discuss it and to talk through all the risks and benefits of all options. Then you can make your informed decision. If everything discussed lines up with what you already thought, then your decision is an easy one.

Remember: The destination may be the same, but it's the journey that matters.

4. I talked to my friend who said ...

Unless your friend is a specialist in the same area as your doctor, don't mention it. Your friend may even have the same condition, but no two people are the same, even if they appear to be. What's right for him or her is not necessarily right for you. Your friend may be exactly right, but this falls in the same category as the previous, "Knowing what you want." Don't demean your doctor by implying your untrained friend knows more than she does. Even if that's not your intention, be careful how you word it. You might be tempted to say, "I spoke to my friend and he said I should try 'X,' and I would like to try it." It's not really a demanding phrase, and it's not aggressive. In fact, it's relatively polite. But by saying that, you imply that you have already made your decision. The doctor has no idea if you are actually informed about X or not. She has a duty to ensure that you are. My recommendation would be to instead try, "I've heard X can be quite effective for (insert your condition). Is this something you might recommend for someone like me? Would you be able to talk me through its benefits and side effects, please?" Even though you may already be informed, it doesn't hurt to have your doctor go over things. She may come up with something you haven't heard before. But the most important thing is that even though you may be informed, you still care what she thinks. You don't have to agree with her, but you should listen.

5. I looked on the internet and ...

I love the internet. I'm just old enough to have been around in the good old days when it emerged and showed the world how powerful of a tool it is, but for every good thing on the web, there's at least an equal number of bad. You know this. If you do research on the internet, make sure you use trusted sources. So instead of saying, "I looked on the internet," say, "I was looking through the literature on 'X's website," providing X is a trusted resource, that is. This will carry more weight than using "the internet." She will have much more faith in a trusted source and will be happier that you are more reliably informed.

So how do you know if your information is from a trusted website? As a general rule, stick with government websites, as well as organizations like the World Health Organization. Other good bets are registered nonprofit charities for your specific condition.

6. Don't quote stats!

Often when we want to reinforce an argument or point of view, we find ourselves reaching for the stats.

This may work in other areas, but healthcare can be fickle. A huge number of patients come and go each day through a doctor's office. Do you really know if you are or aren't that 1 in 10 people that you're quoting?

Stats can also be interpreted in different ways, so they can be difficult to be taken as facts. Things aren't so black-and-white. The authors of a piece of research may interpret it one way, and the whole community may interpret it another. Caution should always be taken when dealing with stats. No piece of research is perfect. There is always an "unless" or a "but."

The chances that you are going to quote a stat that your doctor hasn't heard yet or committed to memory already are quite slim. Of course there are exceptions, and if you've found one, take the advice we've already discussed and don't try to belittle your doctor. Don't be aggressive. Discuss it as peers. Don't argue like children or presidential candidates.

If there is a new piece of research that you really do want to discuss, start by asking if your doctor has already read it. If not, tell her that if she's interested you'll send her a copy, or offer her your copy. Don't say, "Here, I printed you a copy." That could be considered underhanded. Manipulation doesn't breed trust. Next time you see her, you can ask if she read it.

If not, then you can mention your thoughts and conclusions. Don't force it the first time. Let your doctor critique it. You should also see if the research has been reviewed by third-party sources, such as a disease-specific organization or even a national or international organization (think World Health Organization, Department of Health and Human Services or the Department of Health.)

Building the confidence to question your doctor

Not everyone is confident, and even if you are a confident person, you may not be when you get into the doctor's office. The strange thing about confidence is that it can be found in the areas of your life you are an expert in, or at least perceive yourself to be. There is no hack to gaining it, either. Building up confidence takes work and persistence. It's something that has to be earned.

But here's the thing—confidence is empowering. If you want to feel empowered so you can take charge of your healthcare appointments, you have to start with building confidence. It's a must.

Speaking up in a doctor's appointment can be tough. Have you ever found yourself just sitting there and nodding along in agreement, even though you may not understand or agree? If that's you, you're not alone. It's actually quite common.

Confidence and success go hand in hand. If you see someone who is successful, the chances are that person is walking with his or her head held high and exuding confidence. Don't be jealous of that person. That could be you, too. Let's look at what you can do to help improve your confidence.

Do your homework

The one thing that worked for me in the past was making sure I was prepared. Hopefully, if you've gotten this far in the book, you have a good idea how you might achieve that. Planning can help tremendously with your confidence. It's much easier to ask a question if you've written it down first, as you don't have to find the right words and worry about articulating your question. If you're nervous, the words won't come easily, so having them prepared takes that stress away, and the more you do it, the less you'll find yourself relying on that piece of paper in front of you.

Of course this method will only succeed if what you plan to ask is appropriate and well thought-out, which can be hard, especially if you have no idea what you'll be talking about. But if you have a specific problem that needs addressing, there is nothing stopping you from doing plenty of research ahead of time and preparing a list of questions. They don't all necessarily need to be asked. You could easily have one question for treatment option A, one for treatment option B, and so on.

The other upside of doing your research ahead of time is that you are learning. You will be learning more about your condition and its intricacies. Building that knowledge will help you feel more confident over time, and will help you start to feel like an expert, so you will start to hold your head high.

Mastering self-talk

We all have a voice inside of our head that talks to us and lets us know what we are thinking. Mine's called Bob (just kidding).

Self-talk can be limiting and self-defeatist. Have you ever told yourself, "This is hard, I don't think I can do this?" Be honest. I'm pretty sure everyone has said that to themselves at some point. But negative self-talk is damaging to your confidence. It's hard to change it, too, but in order to succeed you need to develop positive self-talk. If you find yourself saying something negative, turn it around and say something positive. Turn the "I'm going to mess this up again" into "I'm going to make it work this time," and then repeat it. The more you repeat it, the more you'll start to believe it.

Stop comparing

Comparing yourself to someone else is never a good thing. You are either going to sink in mood because you feel you're not as good as that person, or you are going to get arrogant because you think you are better than him or her. Either way, you lose. Confidence doesn't come from being better than somebody else. Confidence comes from knowing you are the best you that you can be. Being comfortable in their own skin is what makes confident people confident. You never can truly be at peace with yourself if you are always comparing yourself to others. Instead compare yourself to you yesterday. Are you a better you today than you were yesterday? I hope so.

Diet and exercise

Information about the importance of diet and exercise are everywhere, but do they actually help you feel more confident? Of course they do. Chances are you knew this already. Eat well and your brain will have a steady supply of sugars to keep it active and happy. Eat badly and you'll get sugar spikes, causing highs followed by crashes and low mood. The same goes for exercise. It'll help you maintain your energy levels through the day, making you feel happier in general, which makes it easier to think positively. Exercise also helps stimulate the production of those all-important endorphins, so you can feel happy about yourself for longer. Don't underestimate the effect diet and exercise can have on your mood and confidence.

You're already successful!

Whether you think it or not, you are! Reminding yourself of that fact will help you realize you can achieve your goals. So try this: write down the ten best achievements in your life. It'll be harder than you think. Your achievements can be anything—if you're proud of it, write it down. Nothing breeds confidence more than meeting your goals in life. (Well, actually, maybe being hit on by an attractive partner does. Do you have an attractive partner already? Put it on the list!) Next time you are feeling low or find yourself using negative self-talk, look at the list. It will remind you of all you have achieved so far. The list can only get longer.

Set a goal

Remember that list we just talked about? Let's make it longer. Let's set more goals and achieve them for a boost in confidence. For this, keep the goals small. It will improve your chances of success. That may seem like cheating, but the point isn't necessarily the goal itself (although that is still important). In order to change habits and to reinforce confidence, you need constant reminders that you're awesome, because you are! Smaller, achievable goals will help reinforce that confidence. Now if your goals are too easy, you may find that achieving them has the opposite effect. They still have to be worth achieving, and they don't have to be health-related. We are looking at improving your overall confidence level. Once you achieve one goal, set another. And if you fail, analyze it. Maybe even do a reflective account—see the next chapter— and find out why you failed. And if it's possible, have another go at that same goal. I bet you'll nail it this time.

Build knowledge

When you've set your goal, you may not be sure how you are going to achieve it. It may, in fact, demand you acquire or learn a new skill or skills. Excellent. Learning new things helps us deepen that confidence. How do you know you learned something? You probably passed a test or solved a problem. That means you accomplished something. It may not have been the initial goal, but it's still an achievement. Celebrate it. And if need be, add it to your achievement list.

Recording your appointment

Have you ever had a conversation with someone and then immediately afterwards forgotten what you talked about? Yeah, me, too. And has this ever happened after a doctor's appointment? Yeah, me, too, again. When a lot of information is crammed into a short space of time, it is hard for anyone to remember everything. Of course you should receive a summary of the appointment in some form after your appointment from your doctor, but that will focus on the main aspects of the appointment, and it will be brief and probably full of jargon. Recording the things that are important to you will help you make sure nothing is forgotten.

When it comes to recording the appointment, I've met two types of doctors. Some encourage it, because they want to make sure you understand what is said and that you follow through with action plans. The other type is the suspicious kind, the ones who think you might be using your recording as evidence against them in a future complaint or lawsuit. In my experience, and yours may well be different, neither type minds if you take notes, and I've never seen a doctor ask a patient not to take notes. The second group, the suspicious ones, are only that way because of their own insecurities, making them more likely to make sure that you have a positive appointment, for your benefit and theirs. No one wants a patient to complain, whether it's justified or not.

Regardless which group your doctor or healthcare professional falls into, you should always ask permission first. Always. I'm sure there are random odd cases where a doctor has said no, but 99.99 percent of doctors will not mind. You want to keep a healthy relationship with your doctor, so always ask, even if you have seen her a hundred times. People like being asked. They don't like others to assume it's okay, even if it is. A doctor (should) always ask before examining you, even though it's assumed that it's okay. That's what you're there for, right? But you expect her to ask permission first. I know an examination is more personal and is different from taking notes, but the underlying ethos is the same. People like to be asked.

Now that we have permission, let's look at the "how" and the "what."

How to record your appointment

The most obvious and common way is with a simple notepad and pen. This will serve most people reliably and will be the most comfortable medium to use. There are a few other less common ways, so I wanted to mention those briefly.

The world gets more digital each year, so instead of taking notes on paper and pen you can do it on your phone or tablet using a note-taking app such as Evernote or OneNote. When you ask for permission to take notes, make sure you mention you will be doing so on your mobile device. You don't want your doctor to think you're not paying attention because you're trying to catch Pokémon instead, or because you're checking your email.

The other way is to record the audio for the whole appointment, either with a Dictaphone or with a similar app on your mobile device. This method makes people nervous, and it's not one I usually recommend. You're trying to take positive steps to improve your doctor-patient relationship. Making your doctor nervous usually is not a good way to start. It may also distract your doctor, because she'll constantly be aware that every word she says is being recorded. However, not everyone has the ability to take physical notes. If you have severe rheumatoid arthritis or are an amputee, then this may be the only option available to you. The doctor will understand if this is the case and will be more amenable to audio recordings.

What to record

When making your notes, you should do so in a fashion that suits you. Most people have their own personal shorthand. It doesn't matter, as long as you understand it when you read it back. You shouldn't write down every word. That's counterproductive. Keep your notes brief, using single words or short sentences. The trick to note-taking, of course, is to do so while concentrating on listening, too. It takes time and practice to do both simultaneously. There is no secret trick as far as I know, sorry.

What you should definitely write down is anything you don't understand, whether it be jargon or a concept. This will help you remember to ask the doctor about it later, if you don't at the time. It will also help you when you get home because you can Google (or Bing) the term to get a fuller understanding of it.

I would also recommend writing down any prospective treatments, too. It's better to make sure your insurance covers it before you start, rather than wait until it's already been prescribed. No one likes an unexpected medical bill.

We spoke earlier about taking a list of questions with you to your appointment. You may find your notes will answer some of those for you. If so, great. If not, make sure you write the answers down when you've asked the question! Many times I've had a call from patients saying, "I know I asked earlier, but I don't remember what you said when I asked." That's because they didn't write it down. If you ask a question but don't remember the answer, did you really ask the question? That's one for the philosophers. But I'm going with no, you didn't.

A general rule of thumb should be: If you don't know if you should write it down, then you probably should. Better to be safe than sorry.

Ending your appointment

Without a doubt, the most important part of any appointment is often the most overlooked—the end. The end of the appointment too often is rushed, especially if you ran over the allotted time, or if the clinic as a whole is running late. This is often compounded by the patient feeling overwhelmed by an information-heavy appointment. The result is the "doh!" factor, that feeling when you get home and realize that you forgot to ask something important, or you have no idea what they meant by something. If you've never watched "The Simpsons," you're probably still confused.

So far, you've put in a lot of work, so let's not fall over on the last hurdle. There are things you can do to help you make sure the end of the appointment is as much of a success as the rest. Not all of these will be needed in each appointment, but having an overview will help you make sure your appointment isn't a wasted opportunity. Let's dig into a few of the key points.

Summarize the appointment

Throughout the appointment you have been making notes, hopefully. Now is the time to make sure you didn't miss anything. Go over each point that you wrote to make sure you got everything down, and ask, "Did I miss anything?" It is that simple, but often this is the first step to be skipped in a rush. If you're the kind of person who gets home and thinks, "I knew there was something else, but I can't for the life of me think what it was," then the chances are you skipped this step, or you didn't write anything down.

Revise anything you didn't understand

This is something that can be done as things are said that you don't understand, but sometimes you might not feel like interrupting, nor may it be appropriate to do so. However, it's important that you don't leave with any unanswered questions, particularly if there is unexplained jargon.

When I've spoken to people about their appointments after the fact and they tell me they didn't understand something, of course I ask them, "Why didn't you tell them you didn't understand?" The most common responses I hear are, "I don't know" and "I didn't want to appear stupid." If there is ever a moment for a sitcom-style facepalm, this is it. Those who say "I don't know" deep down do know why, and it was probably because they didn't want to look stupid, and they think admitting that makes them look even more stupid. It's an infinite cycle that does no good.

No doctor that I've ever met will assume you are stupid for asking a question. Doctors want you to leave the appointment understanding what was said, otherwise it was a waste of time for both of you, if not counterproductive. Don't be afraid—doctors don't bite.

What's the plan—and is there a plan B?

Another compelling reason to revise your notes is to confirm you are both on the same page and that you know what the plan is. Knowing what parts of the plan you are responsible for and what parts your doctor is responsible for is key to effectively completing them, right? It isn't always as clear as you may think. The last thing you want is to turn up at the next appointment and realize you forgot something.

So what happens if things don't work out? What if you have a reaction to the new medication? What happens if you get worse? What happens if there is an emergency? There is always a "what if," so make sure you know before you leave what the plan B is. Often plan B is "call me" or "come back to see me." Regardless, you need to know you are both on the same page.

Coming back for more

With chronic illness, there is almost always another appointment. If there is not, and you get discharged from your doctor's care, then I am very happy things are going well for you. Very rarely do people leave appointments not knowing when they need to come back. Doctors are, in general, very good at making sure the patient knows, but it's always good to check if a follow-up appointment is not mentioned.

Say goodbye with a smile

Appointments don't always go well. Sometimes you receive horrible or life-changing news, but you can be assured it isn't done out of spite. Doctors take no pleasure from it, and if you are deeply saddened and distressed, they understand if you're angry toward them. They would rather you weren't, but they get it. If this is not how your appointment went, there is no excuse for rudeness. Being busy isn't an excuse. You can smile and walk out at the same time. Trust me, I've seen it. You can't expect doctors to treat you with dignity and respect if you don't offer them the same courtesy. You started the appointment with a hearty handshake and a smile. End with it, too. A handshake-and-smile sandwich. What could be better?

Write your to-do-list

Okay, so technically this is erroneously placed, because you should do this when you get home, not at the end of the appointment. But very soon after your appointment, while it's still fresh in your head, you should write your to-do list. If there isn't anything new to do, great. Well done. If there is, get it written down somewhere else. Working from your appointment notes is fine, but there's nothing like pinning your to-do-list to the fridge, or on a virtual sticky note on your computer. Wherever and however you choose to do so, make sure you don't forget about it. Put it somewhere you'll see it!

Done that? Yes? Awesome. Now actually follow through! Keep up your end of the deal and stick to the plan you and your doctor have agreed upon. If you have a change of heart or decide you've made a mistake, talk to your doctor first. Don't just disregard it until you see her next, which likely is months away.

CHAPTER SIX

The Reflective Process

What is it?

The Reflective Process (or Reflective Practice) is an important tool used mostly in practice-based professional learning. As a nurse, I used it often, but I believe it can help the patient, too, if applied correctly.

When I started learning about reflective practice, I was dubious. I considered it a bit "wishy washy." In fact, I was rather dismissive of the process, but I did my due diligence anyway because I was being graded on it during nursing school. How wrong I was. By repeating the process over and over, I came to realize just how useful it is, and I even started applying the process in other aspects of my life.

So let's get a definition on the table. "Reflective practice is the ability to reflect on an action so as to engage in a process of continuous learning."[5] The key underlying rationale for reflective practice is that experience alone does not necessarily lead to learning; deliberate reflecting on experience is essential.[6]

How does it help?

Earlier on, I mentioned that this is an ongoing process, and in order to improve your relationship with your doctor, you need to evaluate each visit. The same goes for the tools you used. If you find something you did in you planning to be redundant, then you know that next time you may not need to do it again. Or, more importantly, if something came up you were not prepared for, then you can be better prepared next time.

This will be a hands-on process. By that I mean I don't want you just to think about it. I want this to be a visceral experience. Get a pen and paper and write it all down. Not only does writing help organize those thoughts and feelings in your head, but you can refer back to it when you approach your next appointment. When you plan for an appointment, you should always consider your reflection from the previous appointment. It will help you plan each visit more effectively by concentrating your efforts where they are needed most.

You should also consider keeping all your reflections together. This way you can compare them after each visit and look for themes. You may find the same things come up again and again. The comparison will help you see your progress so you can adjust your planning and implementation accordingly.

How to use a reflective model?

There are many different models you can use for your reflective process. The one I favor, and am most comfortable with, is the Gibbs model.[7] So for the remainder of this chapter I will be using it to demonstrate the implementation. If you'd rather another, then that's cool. There are many, and they are easy to find. Wikipedia has a good list, and so will your favorite search engine.

One reason I like Gibbs' model is because of its handy illustration of the process, which makes it easy to use and to reference. It also clearly demonstrates how reflective practice is a continuous cycle, a constant flow of learning.

This is what it looks like:

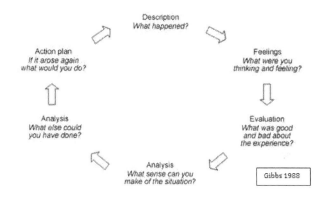

You will find a link to a printable version of this chart in the "Resources" section of this book.

Let's start by splitting up the model into manageable sections, so we can see how it works. The following will include an example reflection to help you further understand how to apply the model:

Description—This simply is describing what happened, without judgment or evaluation. It's just a descriptive sentence or two to get you started.

Feelings—Write these down, but don't analyze them yet. That comes soon. Keep it simple.

Evaluation—Now we start getting into it. This section is about judgments, and listing what was good or bad about the situation or appointment.

Analysis—This is where we try to make sense of it all. Why were the good things good and the bad things bad?

Conclusions (general and specific)—Now give an overall picture of the appointment based on what you analyzed, and not on what you thought before your reflection. They may be different, and that's good.

Action plan—Time to make a plan for what can be done better next time. Make a few actionable goals for the next time you meet. This action plan should be incorporated into your planning for your next appointment.

An example reflection

This is an example of how a reflective account could look. This actually is mostly true—it happened to me, with a few embellishments for the sake of this example only. I hope this helps you with your own reflections.

Description

Saw my rheumatologist for a routine follow-up. Last appointment was three months ago.

Feelings

Anxious about the new pain I'm having in my hip. But also feeling positive that my flare-ups have reduced in frequency since starting my new medication last time.

Evaluation

I have mixed feelings, making it hard to know if it was a good or bad appointment.

> **Good**—The new medication has reduced my flare-up frequency. Both my doctor and I are happy about that. He seems pleased we managed to achieve that.

> **Bad**—My new hip pain was discussed, but I feel like it was overlooked a little. No action was decided on or taken about it. I'm not sure what I need to do, especially if it continues to worsen.

Analysis

The new medication from my last appointment made me feel sick. But he told me it might, so I stuck it out. I'm glad I pushed through and kept to the plan, as the sickness got better as I got used to the medication.

I didn't really ask for any treatment for my hip pain. I assumed it would be offered if there was anything that could have been done. But the last part of the appointment seemed a bit rushed, and that's when I mentioned the hip pain. We spent a lot of time talking about the good news and good changes from the last appointment.

Conclusions (general and specific)

Still feeling ambivalent about my appointment. It seemed to have equal good and bad parts. I think we can do better next time.

Action plan

Mention the problem first or early in the appointment to give time to discuss properly.

Ask if there are treatment options, and which he would suggest.

Research some possible treatments before the appointment, so I have an idea what he might suggest. Will help me make a better decision on the day, without feeling pressured or rushed.

CHAPTER SEVEN

Bringing It All Together

It still amazes me sometimes, the amount of work that we may have to put into a 10-to-15-minute appointment. There's potentially a lot to do beforehand, let alone during and after. If you're feeling overwhelmed now by the amount of information I've thrown at you in a short time, that's okay. There is a lot to remember. I remember feeling overwhelmed once, too. What is important to realize is that this won't all happen in your next appointment. Maybe not even your next ten. It's going to take time to get used to using anything new you have picked up from this book. You shouldn't expect to make it all happen at once. My advice would be to pick one to three new things to do for your next appointment. Start small and build up. Then, at each subsequent appointment, add one more. If you try to do it all at once, you may fail, and that would be disheartening. Build it up slowly, one at a time.

If you can think back to the beginning of this book, you may recall me mentioning picking the right tool for the job. You now have the tools, but please bear in mind that you won't necessarily need them all. Or maybe you'll need to use different ones next year than you did this year. Your health will evolve, and so must your approach and preparation for your appointments. One way of ensuring you evolve your approach is to be guided by your reflections. After all, that's why we do them. They are a learning tool. They will help you learn which tools work best for you. If you use something from this book and it doesn't work for you, that's fine. Feel no obligation to carry on using it. Finding out which tools work best for you sometimes is the hard part, but you will know which work best for you only if you are able to analyze their efficacy.

This book is not a quick-fix guide. No such thing exists. This is a long-term approach to a long-term problem. It's hard to remember that sometimes. Your problems are happening now, which means it's easy for you to concentrate on the present, but keeping one eye on the finish line (your own long-term goal) is imperative to crossing that line successfully.

Otherwise, you run the risk of getting lost on the way and never picking up your winner's medal. There will be roadblocks and detours, but they can be circumvented if you keep an eye on the finish line.

Let's end by celebrating you. Not only do you have impeccable taste in books, but you are unique. Your disease, regardless of how common its prevalence, is unique, too. Remember this often. Healthcare shouldn't take a one-size-fits-all approach. Don't assume that your problems are the same as someone else's and can be "fixed" in the same manner. Neither is true. Your problems are yours and yours alone. That's something to respect. Celebrate your individuality. One of you is all this world can handle, because you're awesome. Remember that often, too.

CHAPTER EIGHT

Resources

To accompany this book, I've created some free resources that you can download and print. These are my gift to you. They are entirely optional. If you have something that works already, or is better for you, use it. These are a guide for those who are struggling or who are new to managing a chronic illness. They also are completely **FREE**. You can alter them to suit you better, if you wish.

There are five resources available. Below is a brief description of each. They are all available to download from my website at http://endlesstrax.com/book-resources/.

You do not have to enter any information to get

them. Just click the download links. You can re-download them anytime, too, should you need.

If you have any questions about using them that aren't already answered in the pages of this book, then please do get in touch.

Also, if you find there is something missing, or a resource you would like, let me know and I'll do my best to get it included for you. You can always email me your feedback at contact@rickywhite.net.

Resources available

Medical Appointments Sheet—Keeping track of your medical appointments can be a challenge. This is a single sheet to help you keep track of them all. It will even help you keep track of whether you have made your next appointment(s).

Symptom History Sheet—Sometimes there are too many symptoms to remember, both past and present. Help keep track of them and of the action you took to resolve them. Don't let any slip through the net and get left untreated.

Medication List Sheet—These days, computers tend to take care of keeping all your medications in one place, but not every healthcare provider is completely digital yet. Or maybe you like doing things the old-fashioned way (I do, too). It's important to list all medications, not just the prescribed ones. Keep them all in one place with this sheet.

Summary Checklist—Finding it hard to keep track of everything you need to do before, during, and after an appointment? Here's a simple checklist to help you make sure nothing is forgotten.

Reflective Model—This is a one-page summary of the Reflective Process. Keep this by your side when you write your reflections. It will help you get a clearer picture of just how your appointment went.

CHAPTER NINE

My Story

The beginning and the misdiagnosis

In keeping with tradition, permit me to start at the beginning. As to when that was, I'm somewhat hazy. That might seem strange to say. Surely I'd remember when I had my first symptoms, but I can't say with accuracy. This in the most part is due to the symptoms themselves. Do you remember the first time you got back pain? Unlikely, because it probably went away for a while. It may have even come back once or twice more, but each time it went away. But after a few times spread over months, or years, you decided maybe you should get it checked out. And being a stubborn young man, I waited until it was at its worst and causing me to miss work. It all started, from what I can recall, in the beginning of 2007, just a year or so into my nursing career.

The problem with ankylosing spondylitis, like many chronic illnesses, is that it often starts with common symptoms, which could have literally hundreds of causes. So with a lack of evidence to prove otherwise, it is misdiagnosed as something more common. That certainly was the case for me. I saw my GP in the United Kingdom several times over the course of a year or so, for what I now know to be flare-ups and the awakening of my illness. Each time it was the same—I had lower back pain and sciatica, so the doctor gave me painkillers. A nurse with lower back pain isn't exactly a rarity. It's almost part of the job description. My managers were amazing (I didn't appreciate it back then), and they sent me to see the occupational health doctor. This is basically a doctor for doctors and nurses. They are employed by the Trust (healthcare provider) to help keep the staff well and productive. My occupational health doctor said something that created a spark that ultimately led me to my correct diagnosis. After my examination, he told me I didn't have chronic back pain. I was too flexible in my lower back, and the physical exam didn't match my symptoms. Instead he told me I most likely had inflammation in my sacroiliac (SI) joint. My sacro-what-now? I was a nurse, but we never covered this in anatomy and physiology class. He briefly explained what it is, and told me it happens sometimes, and that I was best to take anti-inflammatories and try to keep it moving. He referred me for a course of physical therapy. This pattern continued for far too long, and I just kept going along with it.

The unlikely heroes who changed my life

Fast-forward nearly two years, and I had moved to a new job in a new city. After a particularly bad flare-up, I couldn't move without being in extreme pain, and I could hardly walk. I saw my new GP, who said the same as the last. Urgh. Same old. More physical therapy. Then one day, after a few days off sick for another flare-up, I was talking to one of the temporary doctors in the intensive care unit where I worked about my problem. He noticed I'd been off sick (he must have missed me). He was in the Royal Air Force (RAF) and was on a rotation at the time. He said, "I assume they ruled out the serious stuff first, like Ank Spond and stuff?" He wasn't convinced when I replied with something along the lines of "Er ... I assume so." He told me to ask for a special blood test called HLA-B27. I made a mental note. Back then I went to my appointments, sat like a good boy, listened to the doctors, and hoped they knew what they were doing. I wish I could go back and change that. If only I knew what I know now. I never forgot what the RAF doctor had said to me. I wish I could remember his name and rank. I owe him a few beers and a big thank-you.

The next time I went to the doctor I decided I would mention this, and I did. But as luck would have it, I didn't need to. My usual doctor was off sick that day and there was a stand-in doctor covering. She was a young doctor recently out of medical school. Those are the best kind, because they haven't been marred by years of abusive patients and monotonous routine. After I described my problem, she looked up something on the computer. While she was looking, she mentioned doing a blood test—a HLA-B27. I then told her what the RAF doctor had told me, and she said that was exactly what concerned her. Unfortunately, this test took several weeks, because it had to be sent away to a special lab. While I was waiting for the results, I had another flare-up. I saw my regular GP this time, and she was less than pleased that the substitute had ordered such an expensive blood test (it comes from the GP's budget). She said the results were not back yet but that, "if it comes back positive, which I would be surprised if it did," she would refer me to a specialist. She was left to eat her words.

The worst appointment ever and my realization

The consultant rheumatologist I saw on my first appointment was delightful. She confirmed that ankylosing spondylitis was a possibility, but that it was possible to have a positive HLA-B27 test and not to have A.S. (In fact, only one in 15 people who test positive for HLA-B27 go on to develop A.S.[8]) She ordered some X-rays and an MRI scan, and asked me to see her when the results were back. She warned me there was an eight-week wait for non-urgent MRI scans! It was the longest eight weeks ever. I went back for my second appointment for the result and saw who I now assume was the consultant's registrar (her second in command.) But I don't know for sure, because there was no documentation with his name on it! He told me that my scan showed signs of early A.S. but that it was not definite. He said, "If it's not, then it'll go away eventually. If it is ankylosing spondylitis, then your SI joints will fuse together and your pain will go away, so it'll be fine." To this day I cannot repeat those words without getting incredibly angry! He didn't go over treatment with me at all. What I heard from him was, "Deal with it, tough shit," even though those words didn't leave his mouth. Now that I know about A.S., I can tell you that I cannot think of anything worse to say to a patient. At the time, I was in shock. I didn't respond to or question him. When I got home I cried. I cried in anger. Not only was I angry at him, but I was equally angry at myself for just accepting it. Why didn't I say anything? Why didn't I inform myself? What the hell was I playing at? That day changed my life. Without that horrific appointment, I wouldn't be writing this book. A switch was flicked and a fire was started in my belly. No more. I was going to take charge of my health from now on.

The big smoke and my darkest days

Before I could see a rheumatologist again, I got another new job in the big smoke (London). So I packed my bags and moved. I hadn't been there long when I suffered my worst-ever flare-up. I was off work for three months, and it took me around fifteen minutes to walk to the bathroom. It was twenty feet away. Those were my darkest days. I slipped into depression and became reclusive. I have only my wife (who was my fiancée at the time) to thank for getting me through it mentally. I can't thank her enough.

I saw my new rheumatologist at this time. He was a no-nonsense chap, but boy, was he thorough. I got the best care I have ever received from him, not because the first thing he did was "officially" diagnose me, but because he taught me so much. He didn't give me literature to read (which is my only criticism of him), but he taught me by showing me what was actually important and what wasn't. His no-nonsense approach was his filter. He filtered out the irrelevant information, which left him with the core aspects and problems that needed to be addressed. And he was certainly proactive with regard to treatments. He started me on a biologic medication (also called anti-TNF medication) that altered my immune system, immediately. Soon my dark days were over, and I began to realize taking charge of my health and being informed were the best things I could do for myself.

The first step I truly took in taking charge of my health was finding and getting in touch with the National Ankylosing Spondylitis Society (NASS), the United Kingdom's only dedicated ankylosing spondylitis charity. If I have one tip for anyone newly diagnosed, it is to find your local A.S. charity. They will help you more than you would ever think possible and inform you so you can make good, solid choices about your health. The equivalent in the United States is the Spondylitis Association of America.

Acceptance and redirection

One of the hardest parts initially about being diagnosed with a chronic illness is truly accepting it. Knowing that there are things you can no longer do, that you once enjoyed, makes it hard not to get angry. True acceptance is being thankful for the things you still can do and feeling positive about the new things you now get to learn and do.

Learning to accept your condition is not the same as giving in to it. A condition such as A.S. needs to be fought. If you lose motivation and willingness to do so, you'll succumb to it, leaving you in increasingly more pain and becoming more disabled. Unfortunately, this may still happen even if you don't succumb to it, but it would be even worse if you do.

I'm afraid I have no words of wisdom as to how I achieved acceptance; I'm not a psychologist. Maybe it is different for everyone. All I can tell you is that it took me years to truly accept it. Once I did, things started to get a lot easier.

Once I realized that A.S. was a degenerative condition, I knew I'd have to do something about my chosen career path. I was unable to physically manage working on an intensive care unit without causing myself great pain. So I decided to take a sidestep and head in a different direction, to pre-operative assessments. I'm not going to lie: No more night shifts or weekends also had quite an appeal to it. I knew a physically less demanding job, a "desk job," would be a better fit for me. My new job made me realize I had no idea how the system really worked. It was a steep learning curve, to say the least. And that's when it dawned on me that I could use what I learned at work to help me in my own healthcare appointments, because knowing the system helps. And, without me knowing it at the time, the idea for this book was formed.

I spent the next five-plus years trying to do what I could to stay on top of my condition. I didn't always manage it. But each time I failed, I learned. I adjusted and moved on. At one point I had every medication thrown at me, so many that I rattled when I walked, but I somehow felt better off them. With no real improvement in my symptoms, the medications dropped of my list one by one. I saw this as a good thing.

Then came the second-biggest change of my life (the first being fatherhood): We decided to emigrate to the United States. My health and the change in healthcare system certainly was a big consideration, but we decided to go all the same. How exciting!

Crossing the pond

In October 2014, I became an expatriate, leaving behind all my friends and family. It's tough to leave people behind, but at least there is comfort knowing the barriers to staying in touch that once existed no longer do. The internet has been a big help, not only with email but also with video calling.

My first challenge was to master no longer being the breadwinner, and instead taking on the role of the stay-at-home parent. The second challenge was to navigate the new healthcare system. Research will only get you so far—you have to experience it to truly understand it. I'm still working on mastering the new healthcare system and being a stay-at-home dad, but you never know—any day now ...

By using my approach to my doctor's appointment, as I've outlined in this book, I was able to start developing a good relationship with my rheumatologist. Unfortunately, just as I was making good ground, I had to change insurance providers and find new doctors. My new doctors are great, especially my primary care doctor, because I was determined to start off on the right foot so we could develop a positive relationship.

Despite good working relationships with my team of

doctors, my health was not in a good place. It had been far worse, but it had also been far better. One of the hardest parts about being a stay-at-home parent is the close proximity of the fridge. It's always there calling you, asking you to drink sugary drinks and to consume unhealthy snacks. Even before I moved across the pond, my weight had slipped, and now it was even worse. This is a problem in A.S.: More weight means more stress on your joints. It had also been a long time since I worked out, so my core and back muscles were not in good shape. My daily pain levels were gradually rising, and my stiffness and fatigue were worsening. I knew what I had to do, and I knew why. I just needed to find the motivation to do it and to succeed.

Thankfully I found my motivation. It was staring at me with greasy fingers asking for more chicken nuggets. My kids were my motivation. How could I raise them to be healthy, responsible adults if I continued to shirk my responsibility for my own health while I stuffed my face with a greasy hamburger? If I wished to instill these values into my noisy offspring, I would have to lead by example. No one ever learned anything from a hypocrite.

In many ways, the easiest and the hardest part was changing my diet. It's hard to form new habits and to break old ones, but with a strong enough motivation, anyone can do it. So, armed with a new calorie-counting app and a hundred blog posts that contradicted each other about how to eat healthily, I began the task.

The next task was to get into an exercise routine that was a) conducive to my A.S., and b) one that would hold my attention, thus increasing my chances of it becoming part of my lifestyle, rather than a New Year's resolution that I would give up. What I settled on was one of the best decisions I've made in my life. I started training in martial arts again (I had as a child from about 8 to 13 years old). I started training in kempo, or, to be precise, Shaolin kempo.

Clearly not everyone with A.S. is able to train in martial arts, but I think most people have misconceptions about how much they actually can do. Your body, even a diseased one, often can achieve more than you think, and a good martial arts instructor will be able to adjust exercises to meet your needs and to help you achieve your goals. My outcome after eighteen months of training was astonishing. I dropped 30 pounds, and I'm no longer classed as overweight. I've become the fittest, and strongest, I have ever been, especially in my core, which is vital for someone with A.S.

As a result from these two changes in my lifestyle, I

have reduced my medications to a minimum, and some days I have almost no pain. Without any of that, I doubt this book would have come to fruition. I wouldn't have had the energy or concentration because of my pain. If you're interested, you can read the start of my kempo journey here: https://www.potomackempo.com/student-essay-ricky/.

What's important is not what I did to help my health but how I achieved it. Of course eating better and exercising more will help anyone, but I chose to change those two things because they would have the biggest impact on my health. I ignored how hard it would be, because I knew it was achievable. Saying you can't do something before you've tried is foolish. Likewise, not doing something because it's too hard is just as foolish. The hard part isn't the task itself—that can be overcome with good planning and research. The hard part is changing your mindset. Once you've done that, you can achieve what you once considered hard. Pick the most important thing about your illness you can change, and set plans into action to change it. Don't consider how hard it will be; just try. You'll be better for it.

Continual learning

My story hasn't ended yet, thankfully. I hope it will continue for many, many years to come. But for now, I'm in a good place. Settling in a good place makes complacency even more dangerous. I always feel happier when I'm going forward, even if my health isn't. It won't go forward; A.S. is degenerative. The best I can hope for is that my symptoms become stable. But that won't stop me trying to do more to help myself. And despite writing this book, I know that I'll continue to learn. After my dark days I started an A.S. blog, endlesstrax.com. This helped me gain clarity and perspective on my health and being. I realized it was more important to focus on the things I still can do (especially the ones I do well) than it was to look at the things I no longer can do. Grieving over the loss of function, and being made to feel helpless by having something "taken away," no longer served a purpose. I was done defining myself by my condition and by the things I used to do. My perspective, through my writings, changed. I was now defining myself by celebrating what I could do and what I still wanted to achieve. Back then, if you were to ask me to define myself, I would have used words like "nurse" and "ankylosing spondylitis sufferer." Now, if you were to ask me, I would say: "father," "husband," "martial artist," and "bonsai enthusiast." I will also use words that define my work, such as "writer" or "entrepreneur," but they might not even make the top five. My perspective has changed to concentrate on the things that matter to me. If your work truly makes you happy, that's great. But if it doesn't, my advice would be to focus your energy on the things that do make you happy. It may be something already present in your life, or maybe it'll be something you've always wanted to do, like write a book ...

I like quotes. There is pretty much one for everything. But the one that is resonating with me these days is by some chap called Albert Einstein. He (apparently) once said, "Once you stop learning, you start dying." It resonates with me because that's how I approach life now. I always have to be learning something. This is especially true when it comes to my A.S. and managing it. My condition will change and evolve. It already has, so I need to understand why it has, and what I can do to change with it. This might be true for everyone, but I know I will succeed or fail by my ability to adapt to the changes that face me. In order to adapt I need to learn, to keep an open mind, and, most of all, to love myself for who I am and for who I have become. I would implore you to strive to do the same.

CHAPTER TEN

Reference List

1. Ward BW, Schiller JS, Goodman RA. Multiple chronic conditions among US adults: a 2012 update. Prev Chronic Dis. 2014;11:130389. DOI: http://dx.doi.org/10.5888/pcd11.130389

2. Centers for Disease Control and Prevention. National Ambulatory Medical Care Survey: 2012 State and National Summary Tables. http://www.cdc.gov/nchs/data/ahcd/namcs_summary/2012_namcs_web_tables.pdf.

3. Parkinson, CN. (November 19, 1955). "Parkinson's Law". The Economist.

4. Garrett, S; et al (1994). A new approach to defining disease status in ankylosing spondylitis: the Bath Ankylosing Spondylitis Disease Activity Index. Journal of Rheumatology. Dec;21(12):2286-91.

5. Schön, DA. (1983). The reflective practitioner: how professionals think in action. New York: Basic Books.

6. Loughran, JJ. Effective reflective practice: in search of meaning in learning about teaching. Journal of Teacher Education; 2002. 53(1): 33–43.

7. Gibbs, Graham (1988). Learning by doing: a guide to teaching and learning methods. London: Further Education Unit.

8. National Ankylosing Spondylitis Society (NASS). Next steps toward diagnosis, viewed 30 October 2016. http://nass.co.uk/about-as/getting-my-diagnosis/next-steps-towards-diagnosis/.

CHAPTER ELEVEN

Need More Help?

This book has given you some tools you can use to improve your relationship with your doctor, which will ultimately lead to better care, but is it enough for you?

If you've found that you have implemented the advice in this book, downloaded and used the resources, but that you still are feeling unsatisfied with your appointments, what next?

If this is you, then I would like you to get in touch. I am here to guide you if I can. You may also feel like I haven't covered something that you feel is important. If this is the case, please tell me. It may be something that will benefit someone else, too.

If you want to be the first to receive new content, resources, and news on the topic of this book, I encourage you to subscribe to my email list (http://endlesstrax.com/join-the-club/).

Thank you for choosing to buy this book. Your support means the world to me.

Contact Information

Email: contact@rickywhite.net

Blog: http://endlesstrax.com

Twitter: https://twitter.com/endlesstrax

Facebook:
https://www.facebook.com/rickywhitewriter

Instagram: https://www.instagram.com/endlesstrax

About the Author

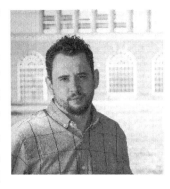

Ricky White is an author based in Virginia, USA. Originally born in Leicester, England, Ricky qualified as a Registered (Adult) Nurse in February 2006. Later he went on to earn his post-graduate degree in Professional Nursing Practice. He worked in a variety of hospitals during his career before he was diagnosed with the chronic, degenerative disease, Ankylosing Spondylitis. Ricky now works as a patient advocate for those with Ankylosing Spondylitis, helping to raise much-needed awareness for his degenerative autoimmune disease.

Because of his unique position in experiencing both sides of the desk, having seen patients in his role as a pre-operative assessment clinic nurse, as well as being a patient himself, Ricky decided to write his debut book — Taking Charge: Making Your Healthcare Appointments Work for You. With the information in this book, Ricky arms other chronic illness sufferers with the tools they need to get the most of their appointments, and to get the care they deserve.

In October 2014, Ricky became a British expatriate

when he moved to Virginia with his wife and children. At this point, Ricky sought to continue his propensity for overworked, underpaid, and underappreciated work by becoming a stay-at-home dad, and he wouldn't have it any other way.

When he is not chasing two under-5-year-olds, he is usually writing, coding, or in the dojo practicing Shaolin Kempo. He also has a mild-moderate addiction to Bonsai trees, of which he has a modest collection.

Ricky can be tracked down between diaper changes via his website – **rickywhite.net**, or on his chronic illness blog – **endlesstrax.com**.

Made in the USA
San Bernardino, CA
19 April 2017